Svante Horsch · Kiriakos Ktenidis
Editors

CURRENT ASPECTS
IN VASCULAR SURGERY

Critical
Limb Ischemia
Carotid Surgery

Diagnosis
and Treatment:

An Interdisciplinary
Approach

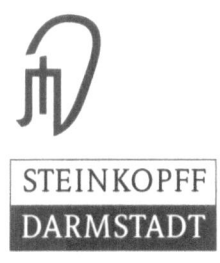

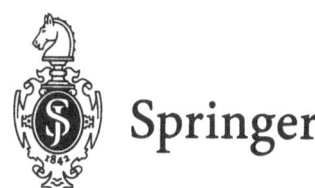 Springer

Editors' addresses:

Prof. Dr. Svante Horsch
Dr. Kiriakos Ktenidis
Krankenhaus Porz am Rhein
Akademisches Lehrkrankenhaus der
Universität zu Köln
Klinik für Allgemeinchirurgie –
Gefäßchirurgie und Traumatologie
Urbacher Weg 19
51149 Köln

Die Deutsche Bibliothek – CIP-Einheitsaufnahme

Critical limb ischemia carotid surgery : current aspects in vascular
surgery ; diagnosis and treatment ; an interdisciplinary approach /
Svante Horsch ; Kiriakos Ktenidis, ed. – Darmstadt : Steinkopff ;
New York : Springer, 1998
  ISBN 978-3-7985-1075-3   ISBN 978-3-642-53788-2 (eBook)
  DOI 10.1007/978-3-642-53788-2

© 1998 by Springer-Verlag Berlin Heidelberg
Originally published by Steinkopff-Verlag Darmstadt in 1998
Softcover reprint of the hardcover 1st edition 1998
Medical Editor: Beate Rühlemann – English Editor: James C. Willis – Production: Heinz J. Schäfer
Cover Design: Erich Kirchner, Heidelberg

Typesetting: Typoservice, Griesheim

Printed on acid-free paper

Foreword

Chronic critical limb ischemia remains one of the most frequent courses of illness and hospitalization in the western world. Interest in critical limb ischemia has increased markedly in recent years. There have been significant achievements in diagnostic procedures as well as in the medical, invasive, and surgical treatment of patients with critical limb ischemia. Dispite considerable research effort, the pathophysiological mechanisms of critical limb ischemia in humans remains to be established.

Prominent is the increasing interest in microcirculation, as well as in the hemorheological, hemostatic, and inflammatory changes which may promote critical limb ischemia.

Further research is necessary to quantify the relevancy of microcirculatory investigations in terms of predicting the prognosis or in evaluating the effects of new therapies.

Our main task is to offer the patients the best possible therapy in order to avoid limb loss and to improve quality of life. The various methods of treatment, their success rates, and their complications must be carefully evaluated and discussed.

This volume presents on one side the complex field of diagnosis and treatment of critical limb ischemia; on the other side the knowledge of cerebral occlusive disease that has accumulated is remarkable, considering that many of the investigative and diagnostic tools have only just been devised. Dispite this unusually brief maturation, cerebral revascularization bas become of age and now ranks with coronary revascularization in frequency and importance.

Surgical invasion of new territory always forces a revision of accepted anatomical beliefs, since direct intervention demands a precision beyond that which was previously adequate. The science of noninvasive diagnosis has grown rapidly, predominantly in the area of disease of the extracranial arteries. The application of digital substraction angiography has likewise detected a vast pool of patients with this occlusive lesion, some of which are still at the asymptomatic stage. Studies of the influence of specific risk factors have also reached considerable precision.

This volume presents a complex field of diagnosis and treatment of both critical limb ischemia and carotid surgery. The diagnosis and treatment involves different specialists including angiologists, interventional radiologists, and vascular surgeons. Individual chapters have been writen by Greek and German experts in the various specialities, who present their own experience.

We are very grateful that these experts have joined us to produce this book.

Finally we would like to thank the publisher, Dr. Dietrich Steinkopff Verlag, for support and assistance.

Cologne, January 1998   Prof. Dr. S. Horsch

Contents

Part II   Carotid Surgery

Critical limb ischemia: definition, incidence and prevalence, pathophysiology and diagnostic management

L. Claeys, K. Ktenidis, S. Horsch

Department of General and Vascular Surgery, Krankenhaus Porz am Rhein, Academic Teaching Hospital of the University of Cologne, Germany

Definition of critical limb ischemia (CLI)

The earliest classification, described by Fontaine in 1950's (1) is based on signs and clinical symptoms, and is very useful in daily practice: stage I, asymptomatic or oligosymptomatic; stage II, intermittent claudication; stage III, ischemic pain at rest (forefoot); stage IV, ulceration or gangrene (inflammatory pain).

However, a more strict definition is necessary for practical clinical purposes and scientific reasons. In the Second European Consensus Document on Chronic Critical Leg Ischemia (2) CLI is defined by the following criteria.

1) Persistently recurring rest pain requiring analgesia for > 2 weeks plus ankle systolic pressure < 50 mm Hg and/or toe systolic pressure < 30 mm Hg; and/or

2) ulceration or gangrene plus ankle systolic pressure < 50 mm Hg and/or toe systolic pressure < 30 mm Hg (absent palpable pulses are sufficient for definition of CLI in diabetes).

Further evidence of ischemia has to be obtained by intraarterial angiography and one of the following tests: a) absence of arterial pulsations in big toe (strain gauge or photoplethysmography); b) assessment of the microcirculation by transcutaneous (Tc) PO_2 (< 10 mm Hg despite O_2-inhalation) and capillaroscopy (morphology and function).

Incidence and prevalence of CLI

There is little information on the epidemiology of CLI. In a review of the literature it is concluded that 1.5 % of men less than 50 years of age and 5 % of men aged over 50 years will have symptomatic leg disease (3). Progressive deterioration of intermittent claudication to rest pain or ulcers/gangrene occurs in ~ 25 % of patients and is estimated to affect 500 − 1000 patients/million population (4). The estimated incidence of major amputations is 120 − 320/million population per year (2). The prevalence of diabetes varies from 2 to 5 %, 10 − 20 % of whom are type I and 89 − 90 % type II (5, 6). The incidence of type I is 4.4 − 29.5/100000 per year, and the incidence of type II 5 − 940/100000 per year.

Prognosis and fate of patients with CLI

The natural history of patients with CLI is known to be bad. According to the experience of the UK Joint Vascular Research Group, approx. 60 % of the patients with CLI will undergo vascular reconstruction, 20 % primary amputation, and 20 % other therapies. One year later 20 % will be dead, 25 % will have had a major amputation. Among the amputees, 50 % will survive for 3 years and only 25 % for 5 years. The other 55 % will have retained both legs (2). Patients with CLI have high mortality and their prognosis is even worse after amputation. The perioperative mortality for below-knee amputation is ~ 5 − 10 %, and for above-knee amputation ~ 15 − 20 %. Long-term mortality ranges from 25 to 30 % 2 years after amputation and 50 − 70 % after 5 years (2). In patients with CLI and diabetes, the risk to develop critical ischemia is five times higher. Among the elderly patients 10 % will develop ulcers or gangrene and the amputation rate is up to 15 times higher. Perioperative mortality is as high as 25 % and only about 50 % alive after 3 years (7).

Pathophysiology of CLI

Atherosclerosis is the fundamental problem in the pathogenesis of CLI. The reduction of the blood flow and perfusion pressure to the distal circulation will cause a flow reduction in the microcirculation. Platelets and leukocytes become activated as they pass over ulcerated plaques, leading to limb perfusion with activated platelets and leukocytes. Decreased capillary perfusion can also result from a combination of venous and arterial insufficiency and a decreased cardiac output may also aggravate limb ischemia.

Different mechanisms are involved in the pathophysiology of the microcirculation: a reduced functional capillary density, a capillary dilatation, a low red cell velocity, microthrombi, abnormal vasomotion, vasospasm, rheological factors, etc. The distribution of the microcirculatory blood flow is regulated by a microvascular flow regulating system (MFRS). A microvascular defence system (MDS), consisting of an interaction between platelets, leukocytes and endothelium, reacts to injury and infection. Prostaglandin I2 is a potent vasodilator and inhibitor of platelet aggregation, which is released from endothelium by mechanical injury or by interaction with platelets or leukocytes and is viewed as being of prime importance in normalising MFRS and deactivating MDS in limb ischemia.

In CLI there is a breakdown of the MFRS and an inappropriate activation of the MDS due to a reduced arterial perfusion (→ maldistribution of blood flow in the nutritive capillaries), an activation of platelets and leukocytes (→ release of vasoconstrictor substances), de-endothelialisation, metabolic changes, release of growth factors and an impairement of blood rheology.

These abnormalities described are further exaggerated in diabetic patients. Furthermore, the autonomic neuropathy complicates the pathophysiology. Diabetic microangiopathy is characterized by a loss of veno-arteriolar reflex, an abnormal vasomotion and an abnormal haemorheology. Immunological and haemorheological factors are also altered and aggravate the vicious cycles in the pathogenesis of limb ischemia. The following abnormalities have been noted (2): glycosylated antibodies, modified function of the antibodies, increased platelet adhesion and aggregation, increased adhesion of blood components to the endothelium, reduced PGI2 production by the endothelium, greater release of oxygen free radicals by leukocytes, lowered fibrinolytic activity, thickening of the capillary basement membrane, reduced EDRF release, reduced erythrocyte deformability, functional microcirculatory abnormalities and increased capillary permeability.

Diagnostic management in patients with CLI

Patients with CLI should be referred to a specialised centre. The following investigations are recommended for all patients with limb ischemia: 1) clinical history and examination (diabetes: neurological testing); 2) resting ECG and chest X-ray (ev. exercise ECG); 3) blood tests and bacteriology; 4) assessment of the macrocirculation (segmental blood pressure, systolic toe pressure, Doppler waveform analysis, Doppler scan of carotids, Duplex scanning, angiography); and 5) assessment of the microcirculation by $TcPO_2$, capillaroscopy and laser-Doppler fluxmetry.

Capillaroscopy is a technique with which the blood filling and morphology of the nutritional skin capillaries can be directly and non-invasively evaluated in clinical practice. It enables us to study directly morphology and dynamics of the nutritional skin capillaries. Density of the capillaries and blood filling can be described. Functional parameters such as red blood cell velocity or permeability can be assessed using special devices or computer programmes. The classification of capillary morphology according to Fagrell has been shown to be very practical for predicting the risk of skin ulcers in patients with CLI; a superior sensitivity and specificity of capillaroscopy was found over systolic toe pressure in prediction of skin necrosis (9).

Laser-Doppler has also been used to study microcirculatory blood flow in patients with CLI. With this method skin perfusion is studied to a penetration depth of 1 mm, and both nutritional and thermoregulatory blood flow are measured. The principle disadvantage is that it is impossible to calibrate in absolute units and that it is very sensitive to artefacts. It is useful for studying the vasomotion in the capillaries. In patients with CLI there may be a reduction in low-frequency motion waves and the appearance of small flux-motion waves with a higher frequency. However, this technique seems not to be useful for predicting the risk of developing skin necrosis.

The transcutaneous oximeter utilizes a Clark-type oxygen-sensing electrode. The heating element of the electrode is warmed to $43-45$ °C, leading to a maximal vasodilation of the microcirculation. $TcPO_2$ is measured with the patient resting in the supine position and the electrodes are attached at the dorsum of the foot and one electrode is attached at the chest in order to obtain a reference value. The ratio between limb and chest $TcPO_2$ is referred to as the regional perfusion index. Modifications of this technique are $TcPO_2$-measurement under oxygen inhalation and the measurement of the postocclusive limb $TcPO_2$ recovery time. Stress testing can be performed in elevating the leg to 30° for 3 min.

Transcutaneous oximetry is useful for diagnosing and localizing critical ischemia of the limbs, in determining the severity of the disease, in predicting the amputation level and as non-invasive method in studying microcirculatory function. However, many physiological, methodological and technical factors influence the measurements and this limits the value of $TcPO_2$ data.

Conclusion

The definition of CLI proposed in the Second European Consensus Document on Chronic Critical Leg Ischemia is based on strict criteria and very useful in daily practice. However, further evidence of ischemia has to be obtained by the study of the microcirculation. The relevance of microcirculatory measurements should be quantified by prospective studies, analysing the specificity/sensitivity in terms of predicting prognosis. Epidemiological studies are necessary to obtain more detailed data concerning the incidence, prevalence and prognosis of CLI. Of special interest is the degree of reversibility of the patho-physiological changes under different therapies.

References

1. Fontaine R, Dubost C (1954) Les greffes vasculaires. Rapport au Congrès de Chirurgie, Paris
2. Second European Consensus Document on Chronic Critical Leg Ischemia (1991) Circulation 84: 1–21
3. Fowkes FGR (1988) Epidemiology of atherosclerotic arterial disease in the lower limbs. Eur J Vasc Surg 2: 283–291
4. Lasila R, Lepäntalo M, Lindfors O (1986) Peripheral arterial disease – natural outcome. Acta Med Scand 220: 295–298
5. Krone W, Müller-Wieland D (1990) Special problems of the diabetic patients. In: Dormandy J, Stock G (eds) Critical leg ischemia. Its pathophysiology and its management. Springer, Berlin Heidelberg, pp 145–157
6. Ross H, Rifkin H (1987) Diabetes mellitus: an overview. In: Brenner MA (ed) Management of the diabetic foot. Williams & Wilkins, Baltimore, pp 3–7
7. Krolowski AS, Warram JH (1991) Epidemiology of diabetes mellitus. In: Marble A, Krall LP, Bradley RS, Christlieb AR, Soulidner S (eds) Joslin's diabetes mellitus. Lea & Ferbiger, Philadelphia, pp 12–42
8. Lowe G (1990) Pathophysiology of critical leg ischemia. In: Dormandy J, Stock G (eds) Critical leg ischemia. Its pathophysiology and its management. Springer, Berlin Heidelberg, pp 17–38
9. Fagrell B, Lundberg G (1984) A simplified evaluation of vital capillary microscopy for predicting skin viability in patients with severe arterial insufficiency. Clin Physiol 4: 403–411
10. Tonessen KH (1978) Transcutaneous oxygen tension in imminent foot gangrene. Acta Anaesth Scand 68: 107–110

Author's address:
L. Claeys, MD
Dept. of Vascular Surgery
General Hospital Cologne-Porz
Urbacher Weg 19
51149 Cologne, Germany

Intraoperative thrombolysis as an adjunct to surgery in acute arterial occlusion

J. Dayantas

Department of Vascular Surgery, Athens General Hospital, Athens, Greece

The introduction of the baloon-tipped catheter by Fogarty et al. (1) in the treatment of acute limb ischcmia resulted in improvement both in amputation and mortality rates. However, the excellent results achieved by this method at the early years proved less satisfactory in recent years mainly because of two reasons: firstly, embolic events originate from atherosclerotic heart disease rather than rheumatic as the latter has declined (2, 3) involving advanced age population with associated peripheral arterial disease complicating their management (4). Secondly, a substantial proportion of patients with acute leg ischemia have arterial thrombosis secondary to arteriosclerosis and balloon catheter embolectomy alone is associated with lower limb salvage and higher mortality rate (5, 6).

Balloon catheter embolectomy also fails to remove thrombi from side branches or distal arteries. By angiography, residual thrombi are noticed over 40 per cent of patients (7). Intra-arterial thrombolytic therapy may clear all thrombi in arterial tree even those of embolic origin but may take time jeopardising the viability of acute ischemic limb. Thus, balloon catheter thromboembolectomy remains the treatment of choice in patients presenting with acute ischemia severe enough to cause motorsensory dysfunction.

A solution to overcome the above-mentioned problems is to combine balloon catheter embolectomy with intraoperative thrombolysis (8, 9). By this combination, success rates as high as 100 per cent have been reported (10, 11). The agents used include streptokinase, urokinase and recombinant tissue plasminogen activator (rt-PA). Secondary procedures such as balloon angioplasty and vascular reconstruction may become necessary to correct other underlying lesion at the time or subsequent to lytic therapy (12).

Patients and methods

From January 1992 to December 1994, 237 patients with acute limb ischemia were operated in the Vascular Department of Athens General Hospital. Amongst them there were 14 men and 2 women consisting the present group of patients to whom the combined therapy of balloon catheter thromboembolectomy and intraoperative thrombolysis was applied. The patients age ranged from 27 to 71 years (mean 54). Two were diabetics and one was hypertensive well controlled.

The aetiology of ischemia was femoral/popliteal thrombosis 11, popliteal aneurysm thrombosis two, popliteal entrapment one and embolism two. Two additional cases of popliteal artery trauma with postreconstruction distal ischemia underwent thrombolysis without success but are excluded from this study. The duration of ischemia ranged from 4 to 19 hours (mean 7 h). No contraindications for thrombolysis were present as defined by previous reports (12, 13, 14). Preoperative arteriography was not performed. The ankle/

brachial index measured by Doppler ranged between 0.0 to 0.21 (mean 0.12). Preoperative laboratory evaluations included routine blood tests plus base line coagulation values (prothrombin time, activated partial thromboplastin time, fibrinogen, fibrin split products). In every patient a bolus of 5000 units of heparin was administered on admission and balloon catheter embolectomy was performed in the usual manner. Following balloon thromboembolectomy as well as popliteal aneurysm reconstruction, inadequate back-bleeding or persistent ischemia as determined by physical and Doppler examination were indications for thrombolysis. An intraoperative arteriogram, although no routine in our department was performed and a catheter was introduced with the tip close to the origin of the thrombus.

An initial bolus of 5 mg rt-PA (Actilyse, Boehringer Ingelheim) was infused and following 10 − 15 minute period another pass was made with the balloon catheter. Another arteriogram was obtained and if residual thrombi were noticed the same procedure was repeated. Subsequent embolectomy and 2.5 mg rt-PA infusions were administered to five patients up to two times a total of 15 mg rt-PA. In four patients intra-arterial infusion of 20 − 40 mg Naftidrofuryl oxalate was also administered. All patients maintained on heparin and started oral anticoagulation postoperatively. In two patients, embolectomy and thrombolysis failed to restore distal normal blood flow as revealed by angiography. All patients tolerated the procedure well.

Results

Sixteen patients with acute limb-threatening ischemia were treated by balloon catheter thromboembolectomy and intraoperative thrombolysis with rt-PA. There was neither mortality not serious bleeding complication. Fourteen out of sixteen interventions resulted in clinical restoration of perfusion to the affected limb. Two patients with failed procedure underwent subsequent amputation one above and the other below the knee. In these two patients angiography demonstrated failure to restore distal runoff. Palpable pulses were present in eight from fourteen salvaged limbs. A significant increase was seen in the ankle/brachial index which ranged from 0.3 to 0.8 (mean 0.6). No patient had fibrinogen levels below 100 mg %. Two patients with compartment syndrome underwent fasciotomies. Dosage of rt-PA ranged between 10 to 15 mgs.

Conclusions

Balloon catheter thromboembolectomy remains the treatment of choice in severe acute limb ischemia.

In selected cases intraoperative thrombolysis is a useful and safe additional procedure if distal perfusion cannot be restored by embolectomy alone.

References

1. Fogarty TJ, Cranley JJ, Krause RJ, Strasses FS, Hafner C (1963) A method for extracting arterial emboli and thrombi. Surg Gynecol Obstet 2: 241−4
2. Darling RC, Austen WC, Linton RR (1967) Arterial embolism. Surg Gynecol Obstet 124: 106
3. Abbott WM, Maloney RD, McCabe CC (1982) Arterial embolism: a 44 year perspective. Am J Surg 143: 460
4. Tawes RL, Harris EJ, Brown WH et al. (1985) Arterial thromboembolism: a 20 year perspective. Arch Surg 120: 595−9
5. Humphries AW, Young JR (1970) The severely ischemic leg. Curr Probl Clin Surg 6: 3−59
6. Jivegard L, Holm J, Schersten T (1986) The outcome of arterial embolism misdiagnosed as arterial embolism. Acta Chir Scand 152: 251−6
7. Plecha FR, Pories WT (1972) Intraoperative angiography in the immediate assessment of arterial reconstruction. Arch Surg 105: 902−7
8. Norem RF, Short DH, Kerstein MD (1988) Role of intraoperative fibrinolytic therapy in acute arterial occlusion. Surg Gynecol Obstet 167: 87−91
9. Garcia R, Saroyan MR, Senkowsky J, Smith F, Kerstein M (1990) Intraoperative intra-arterial urokinase infusion as an adjunct to Fogarty catheter embolectomy in acute arterial occlusion. Surg Gynecol Obstet 171: 201−5
10. Quinones-Baldrich WJ, Zierler RE, Hiatt JC (1985) Intraoperative fibrinolytic therapy: an adjunct to catheter thromboembolectomy. J Vasc Surg 2: 319−26
11. Cohen LH, Kaplan M, Bernhard VM (1986) Intraoperative streptokinase: an adjunct to mechanical thrombectomy in the management of acute ischemia. Arch Surg 121: 708−15
12. Comereta AJ, Rubin RN, Tyson RR, White JV et al. (1987) Intra-arterial thrombolytic therapy in peripheral vascular disease. Surg Gynecol Obstet 165: 1−8
13. Dacey LT, Dow RW, McDaniel MD et al. (1988) Cost-effectiveness of intra-arterial thrombolytic therapy. Arch Surg 123: 1218−23
14. Berridge RHS, Gregson BR, Hopkinson, Makin GS (1989) Intra-arterial thrombolysis using recombinant tissue Plasminogen Activator (rt-PA): the optimal agent at the optimal dose? Eur J Vasc Surg 3: 327−32

Author's address:
J. Dayantas
Department of Vascular Surgery
Athens General Hospital
154 Messogion Ave.
11527 Athens, Greece

Percutaneous transluminal angioplasty of the iliofemoral level

D. Mourikis

Department of Radiology, Areteio Hospital, Athens, Greece

The section of Invasive Radiology in Areteio Hospital, Athens University, Diagnostic Radiology Dept., has been developing sinse 1975.

Along with the application of other invasive techniques, angioplasty was introduced in 1980, and it was further developed after 1984 when a digital angiography unit was acquired.

The section of invasive radiology is part of the Diagnostic Radiology Dept. and its main task is angiography and invasive techniques application as well as teaching mainly of radiologists and fourth and sixth year medical students.

The rapid development of the section is greatly due to coexistence in Areteio Hospital of the Vascular Surgery Clinic, which mainly supplies patients from the outpatient pooling, and scientific collaboration with vascular surgeons.

In the last 15 years, 1258 transluminal angioplasty procedures were performed, of which 995 were iliac arteries cases.

Suitable patients for angioplasty are selected in collaboration with surgeons from the outpatients pooling of the Hospital.

Admittance to the hospital is on a 24-h basis. The patients to be selected, apart from clinical evaluation and Doppler examination, also have a digital angiogram.

When strong indication exists the patient is scheduled for intraarterial angiography followed by angioplasty in one step.

Biochemistry and blood tests are included in the preoperative study and blood matching for transfusion in the case of major complication. Cardiac evaluation is not usually mandatory.

Three days prior to angioplasty the patient is given 300 mg of aspirin per day. The patient is usually fasted and prepared in condition vascular surgery will be needed.

Unilateral approach to the site of obstruction is usually performed, or in case of great difficulty, the approach is performed from the oposite femoral or the auxillary artery.

The passage through the stenosis is achieved using the appropriate guidewires, catheters and ballons for each different case. We have not yet used newer technologies like laser and atherotomy devices.

Depending on the texture, the site and the extent of the plaque, we use one or two balloons. Bilateral paracentesis is needed in cases of aortic stenosis or bilateral common iliac

Table 1.

	Number of patients	Solitary stenosis	Multiple stenosis	Occlusions
Illiofemoral arteries	995	735 (95 stents)	112 (8 stents)	45 (14 stents)

stenosis and bilateral balloons are used (kissing balloons). In this manner the contralateral iliac artery is well preserved from possible infarction. Immediately after the use of balloon, the use of metallic stent in iliac arteries is decided. Our main experience is based on Palmaz stents as they give better result in time, with less endothelization in relation to other stents. In cases with torturous vessels with extended stenosis, we use the Schneider self-expandable stents.

Often, angioplasty is performed in iliofemoral bypasses in coordination with local thrombolysis or when stenosis is noted at the site of anastomoses.

Some ilio-femoral angioplasties are performed prior to surgery in order to increase the blood flow to periphery.

The patients are evaluated in 6 month intervals for the first year by Doppler and digital angiography and thereafter every year if clinically indicated. The 5-year follow-up study of 325 patients who underwent iliofemoral PTA shows a 53 % good result of those who had a single balloon angioplasty, and a 71 % good result in patients with a stent placement.

An important factor in the application of the invasive techniques is the organization of the department of digital angiography respective personnel and technical material and equipment. It is evident that the close collaboration with vascular surgeons is needed during angioplasty. In every case of balloon angioplasty there is an operation room available and ready, and the vascular surgeon and the anesthesiologist are very well informed.

The patient and his family are briefed on possible complications.

In conclusion, ilio-femoral angioplasty is today a well established method without major complication or risk.

The collaboration of radiologist and vascular surgeon is essential in the pre- and post-treatment period and the method is assumed to be the gold standard procedure in iliofemoral stenotic lesions.

Author's address:
Prof. D. Mourikis, MD, PhD
Department of Radiology
Areteio Hospital
15, V. Hepeirou Str.
Filothei – Athens, Greece

Complications during and after percutaneous transluminal angioplasty (PTA) of iliac and peripheral arteries

D. Beyer, Ch. Kaiser, M. Kress, S. Horsch

Department of Diagnostic and Interventional Radiology, Krankenhaus Porz am Rhein, Academic Teaching Hospital of the University of Cologne, Germany

In the 30 years since Dotter's and Judkin's original publication (7) of percutaneous trans-luminal dilatation of narrowed or occluded arterial segments, there has been a tremend-ous increase in the number of patients treated using this technique (4). The advantages of PTA include reduced morbidity and mortality as well as the fincancial benefits of reduced in-patients costs, allowing a greater number of patients to undergo this treatment (2). But in the initial enthusiasm for a new method the mostly good clinical and technical results are reported, while minor or severe complications are often disregarded (3).

The literature on PTA has been overwhelming during the past 30 years (1–14). Compli-cations are, however, usually not reported in detail, and relatively few articles are dealing exclusively with the analysis of complications in large series of patients undergoing PTA of iliac and lower extremity arteries. Many authors have commented on the difficulty of com-parison between such studies, as the results reflect not only differing populations and operator experience, but may also involve the use of differing reporting criteria (11).

Reviews concerned with ilio-femoral-popliteal PTA showed complication rates of 11.4 % (Casarella, 1986: 3204 patients), 8.6 % (Weibuhl et al., 1987: 2043 patients), and 2.3 % (requiring surgery) (Zeitler et al., 1983: 1942 patients). Most publications are only case reports (3). Most of these complications (Table 1) are already recognized during the procedure or during arterial compression at the end of the angioplasty.

When dealing with PTA, the radiologist should always remember the old surgical aphorism that there is no such thing as a "little procedure"; even a low-risk procedure can lead to a catastrophic complication (1, 6, 9).

Basic contraindication to peripheral PTA is the availability of a surgical procedure that offers a significant advantage over angioplasty in much the same way that the availability of PTA is a strong contraindication to a more complex or more risky surgical procedure (1).

It must be stressed that there should be a close and confidential cooperation between the department of radiology performing PTA and vascular surgery in the daily care of these patients especially in the treatment of complications of PTA. Therefore the vascular surgeons of our hospital are an important part of the decision process and we treat only patients of this department with PTA. These vascular surgeons on the other hand treat many patients with acute complications of PTAs performed in other hospital departments or out-patient clinics (6, 9).

Interventional radiologists and vascular surgeons of our hospital sign a consent form before PTA demonstrating how and when a patient should undergo this procedure.

We reviewed 836 ilio-femoral-popliteal PTAs (1990 – 1994) performed in our depart-ment intending to discuss methodologic points, analyze various types of complications and show how to avoid and treat them in cooperation with vascular surgeons.

Definition of complications

The scientifically proper way is to define complications before PTA then to analyze their number and clinical consequences prospectively. We considered it important to separate complications occurring at the puncture site and at the dilatation site as well as distant and general complications.

It is also valuable to separate major complications with real clinical implications and consecutive surgery from those which only give a small discomfort or those which are solely seen radiographically (Tables 1, 2).

Analysis of complications

The complications in PTA may occur at different levels: at the puncture site, at the dilatation site, distal from the dilatation site and there are general and radiologic complications.

From a practical point of view each level is analyzed separately.

Complications at puncture site

Major groin hematomas after withdrawal of the balloon catheter are rather common. Small hematomas are usually not reported and the quantification may be difficult. In our series we had two major hematomas, which required surgical treatment (0.24 %).

One reason for hematoma formation was the use of large catheters up to 7F in the first year. Today we mostly use 5F catheters.

Ruptured balloons (n = 13; 1.55 %) have an umbrella-shaped widening making it difficult to withdraw it from the artery through the puncture hole. Modern and Olberttype of balloon catheters have less of these problems, because the balloon after exsufflation is closer to the catheter wall.

Our use of aspirin or heparin in connection with PTA may prolong bleeding time and in combination with a large puncture hole, the risk of developing hematoma may increase. Careful compression over 30 min and frequent control of the puncture site after PTA in our patients were very important. Furthermore, such hematomas can often be prevented by simple, careful instruction of the patient during puncture site compression. Patients need to be told in simple terms that they have to stay in bed for 24 h and to avoid certain activities such as sitting, unaided head rising, or movement of the limb bearing the puncture site.

Infection of the puncture site did not occur in our series. Nevertheless, surgery at the percutaneous catheterization site within the first 5 days carries an elevated risk of local infection. Since the morbidity and mortality resulting from graft infections is high, careful consideration should be given to the timing and location of proposed vascular surgery in planning the vascular approach for PTA.

Table 1. Principal Complications of PTA

I.   **Puncture Site Complications**
  – Arterial dissection
  – Arterial occlusion
  – Hematoma
  – Pseudoaneurysm
  – Arterio-venous fistula formation
  – Nerve damage
  – Infection

II. **Angioplasty Site Complications**
  – Arterial dissection
  – Side branch occlusion
  – Perforation and rupture
  – Arterial spasm
  – Arterio-venous fistula formation
  – Acute or early (in first 24 hours) occlusions
  – Peripheral embolisation

III. **Equipment Complications**
  – Balloon rupture
  – Foreign body embolization (guidewire coating)
  – Difficult catheter removal

IV. **Systemic Complications**
  – Contrast media reactions
  – Contrast media induced renal failure
  – Sepsis

Table 2. Complications of PTA (n = 836)

Major Complications		
Acute Occlusions at PTA-Site	2	(0.24 %)
Early Occlusions (first 24 h after PTA)	4	(0.48 %)
Peripheral Embolism with Consecutive Surgery or Lysis	6	(0.72 %)
Groin Hematoma (with consecutive surgery)	2	(0.24 %)
Ballon Rupture		
– with vessel perforation and local hematoma	1	(0.12 %)
– with vessel perforation, local hematoma and consecutive venous thrombosis	1	(0.12 %)
– with vessel perforation, local hematoma and small pseudoaneurysm	1	(0.12 %)
Acute Contrast Media Reaction	1	(0.12 %)
Late Contrast Media Reaction	1	(0.12 %)
	19	(2.28 %)
Minor Complications		
Non-occlusive Dissection	41	(4.90 %)
Arterial Spasm	26	(3.10 %)
Emotional Problems of the Patient	4	(0.48 %)
Groin Hematoma without Consecutive Surgery	12	(1.44 %)
Minimal Peripheral Embolism without Surgery or Lysis	9	(1.08 %)
	92	(11.00 %)
Equipment Complications		
Balloon Rupture without Vessel Perforation	13	(1.55 %)
Guidewire Coating Problems	2	(0.24 %)
	15	(1.79 %)
Total	126	(15.07 %)

Complications at the dilatation site

Arterial ruptures or perforations as a consequence of balloon dilatations fortunately are very rare. We saw only three perforations (0.36 %) after a balloon rupture with a minute hole in the arterial wall and small local hematomas. In one of these cases we demonstrated the formation of a small pseudoaneurysm at the perforation site after 3 months. In the other case the local hematoma compressed the femoral vein with consecutive venous thrombosis. In case of vessel rupture it is important to keep the balloon catheter in place and, by expanding it, to prevent unnecessary bleeding.

Intimal flaps (non-occlusive dissections) may be seen radiographically at the dilatation site. In our material such small flaps were seen in 41 patients (4.9 %). These flaps as a sign of focal non-occlusive dissection were not of clinical importance, but merely an expression that the dilatation was effective. We think that focal dissection is actually an integral part of the mechanism of angioplasty and thus desirable; the simple presence of an angiographically demonstrable dissection following PTA is not a true complication.

In one case the dissection flap became so extensive that it acted like an occlusive flap valve and caused an early occlusion in the first 24 h after PTA.

If the guide wire had been left across the lesion or the lesion could be easily but carefully retraversed, we "glued" the flap to the vessel wall by a long, 2 – 4 min low-pressure inflation of the balloon. Today, we treat a flow-limiting dissection following an otherwise technically successful PTA especially in the iliac arteries by implanting an endovascular stent (Palmaz type).

Acute (during PTA) *or early occlusions* of dilated segments (in the first 24 h) are reported in a relatively high frequency. In our material this was seen in six cases (0.72 %). After continuous use of 20000 i.u. of heparin in the 24 h following balloon dilatation of the femoral and popliteal arteries additional to the 5000 i.u. of heparin during the procedure we saw only four early occlusions (0.48 %) in the first 24 h after PTA.

Distal complications

Arterial spasms may be caused by the manipulation of guide-wires or catheters in femoral, popliteal or more distal arteries, mostly in young patients. This was seen in 26 PTAs (3.1%). When spasms occurred, intraarterial injections of lidocain, nitroglycerin or calcium blockers such as verapamil and prostavasin were effective and peripheral parenchymal damage did not occur.

Distal macroembolisations with consecutive lysis or surgery, a feared complication of PTA, occurred in six patients (0.72 %) more often after PTA of occlusions than after PTA of stenoses. One large embolus had to be removed surgically with a Fogarty catheter. In five cases we tried to disintegrate the thrombi with administration of urokinase and restitute peripheral perfusion.

General complications

In our series there were no *septic complications* indicated by septic fever and/or positive blood cultures. There were no patients with *renal insufficiency* after PTA. All our patients referred to PTA were well hydrated before, during and after the procedure and the amount of non-ionic contrast media (Ultravist 300) was kept at a minimum. *Allergic contrast media reactions* were seen in two patients (0.25 %) with one acute and one late reaction.

Conclusions

The complication rates of PTA, particularly the technical ones, decrease with time and increasing experience.

In our series of 836 ilio-femoral-popliteal PTAs (1990 – 1994) performed in our department, major and minor complications decreased during the 5 years of increasing experience. There were no limb amputations directly following PTA. Many complications – for instance peripheral spasms, peripheral macroembolization or acute/early vessel occlusions following PTA – are still hard to foresee or to avoid. Re-thrombosis of occlusions in the femoral or popliteal arteries decreased significantly after establishing systemic heparinization following the procedure. Furthermore, careful patient selection in cooperation with the referring vascular surgeons of our institution (consent form!) is very important for a low complication rate. When a complication occurs, surgical backup and immediate surgical intervention may avoid further major damage to the patient. The availability of this emergency care must be fully understood by the patient because there may be an occasional serious delayed complication. Therefore, close cooperation between interventional radiologists and vascular surgeons cannot be too frequently stressed.

In patients with intermittent claudication, our low complication rate justifies the use of PTA, especially if it is possible to treat these complications as a part of the PTA procedure. The low incidence of complications needing surgical intervention does in our belief justify the use of PTA in patients not being considered for reconstructive vascular surgery. This applies to both ends of the clinical spectrum, such as those patients with threatened limb loss and coexistent medical conditions rendering them unfit for major operation, and those who have intermittent claudication due to stenoses which is limiting their activities in work or leisure, but which is not considered severe enough for vascular surgery.

References

1. Ahn SS, Moore WS (1992) Endovascular Surgery. WB Saunders Company, Philadelphia
2. Anderson JB, Wolinski AP, Wells IP, Wilkins DC, Bliss BP (1986) The inpact of percutaneous transluminal angioplasty on the management of peripheral vascular disease. Brit J Surg 73: 17–19
3. Bergquist D, Jonsson K, Weibuhl H (1987) Complications after percutaneous transluminal angioplasty of peripheral and renal arteries. Acta Radiol 28: 3–10
4. Belli AM, Cumberland DC, Knox AM, Procter AE, Welsh CL (1990) The Complication Rate of Percutaneous Peripheral Balloon Angioplasty. Clin Radiol 41: 380–383
5. Casarella WJ (1986) Non-coronary Angioplasty. Curr Probl Cardiol 11: 138–174
6. David A (1993) Gefäßchirurgische Therapie von Komplikationen nach perkutaner transluminaler Angioplastie (PTA). Inaugural-Dissertation Köln 19. 02. 93
7. Dotter CT, Judkins MP (1964) Transluminal treatment of arteriosclerotic obstruction; description of a new technique and a preliminary report of its application. Circulation 30: 654–670
8. Fraedrich G, Beck A, Bonzel T, Schlosser V (1987) Acute Surgical Intervention for Complications of Percutaneous Transluminal Angioplasty. Eur J Vasc Surg 1: 197–203

9. Horsch S, David A, Beyer D (1991) Komplikationen nach perkutaner transluminaler Angioplastie und ihre gefäßchirurgische Therapie. Zent Bl Chir 116: 627–639
10. Lemarbre L, Hudon G, Coches G, Bourassa MG (1987) Outpatient Peripheral Angioplasty: Surgery of Complications and Patient Perceptions. AJR 148: 1239–1240
11. Morse MH, Jeans WD, Cole SEA, Grier D, Ndlovu D (1991) Complications in percutaneous transluminal angioplasty: relationship with age. Brit J Rad 64, 757: 5–9
12. Seyferth W, Ernsting M, Grosse-Vorholt R, Zeitler E (1983) Complications during and after percutaneous transluminal angioplasty. In: Dotter CT, Grüntzig A, Schoop W, Zeitler E. Percutaneous Transluminal Angioplasty, Springer Verlag, Heidelberg Berlin
13. Weibuhl H, Bergquist D, Jonsson K, Karlson S, Takolander R (1987) Complications after percutaneous transluminal angioplasty in the iliac, femoral and peripheral arteries. J Vasc Surg 5: 681–686
14. Zeitler E, Richter E, Roth FJ, Schoop W (1983) Results of percutaneous transluminal angioplasty. Radiology 146: 57–60

Author's address:
Prof. Dieter Beyer, MD, PhD
Department of Diagnostic and Interventional Radiology
Krankenhaus Porz am Rhein
Urbacher Weg 19
51149 Köln, Germany

Vascular surgical interventions required after complications caused by percutaneous transluminal angioplasty PTA

S. Ricke, B. Oehm, K. Heye, S. Horsch, D. Beyer

Department of General and Vascular Surgery, Krankenhaus Porz am Rhein, Academic Teaching Hospital of the University of Cologne, Germany

In the time period January 1986 until April 1995 54 patients were sent to our hospital for further treatment after PTA procedure. 41 of these patients came from foreign hospitals and 13 patients had been treated with a PTA in our own radiological department. Of the mentioned 54 patients, 36 were women and 18 were men with an average age of 49 to 86 years. A high-risk group was not age linked, however, almost all patients had indulged in nicotin over years, suffered from hypercholesterolaemia or had noticed claudication over a number of years.

Results

A good prognostic indicator seems to be the time elapsed between the occurence of post-interventional complications and the additional surgical intervention in our patient group. 31 patients presented immediately, that is within six hours of a complication being noticed, and of these, 13 patients came from our own radiological department. These patients obviously had the advantage of being an in patient and still being under close observation after the radiological intervention. 9 cases presented after a time-interval of about one week. 14 patients were unfortunate enough to only suffer more noticeable complications in a time span of three months up to one year after PTA. The vascular surgical interventions required could be grouped into the following: 20 patients received emergency surgery for either life- or limb-threatening complications. 13 patients required fairly prompt treatment, but did not require emergency surgery. 21 patients received elective surgery.

What were the complications requiring surgical intervention?

These complications were associated with the puncture site in the artery as well as the vessel dilatation more distally. 37 patients had a thrombembolic event. A dissection at the dilatation site occurred in 14 patients. 2 patients had large hematomas with consecutive surgically treatment. The rare occurrence of a thrombosis at the puncture site was described in 3 cases, in all of which a PTA of the contralateral common iliac artery had been successfully completed. Further rareties of complications that we picked up were:

– Development of a foreign spontaneus aneurysm at the puncture site, in one case and

– Development of a foreign body embolisation in the common femoral artery which was identified as the hydrophilic coverage of a lead wire required for dilatation.

We noticed complications in the following arterial systems:
– Aorto once,
– 12 times in the iliac arteries,
– 24 times in the femoral arteries,
– 7 times in the popliteal arteries,
– 7 times in the region of the arterial trifurcation of the lower leg,
– 2 in a renal artery.

It was shown that with the number of complications mentioned, the same patient could suffer lacerations to the vascular system at numerous levels. The patients treated with additional vascular surgery in our hospital received the following operations:

2 patients required an aorto-renal bypass, 1 patient received aorto-iliac bypass, 4 patients required an aorto bi-femoral Y-prosthesis and an ilio-femoral bypass operation was necessary in 3 patients. Most of the patients (21) received a femoro-popliteal bypass as reconstructive measure. 16 patients needed a thrombembolectomy, 1 patient was treated by femoro-crural bypass. Only 1 patient required individual attention: a short-distance graft interposition of the superficial femoral artery, 1 patient required resection and graft interposition of a common femoral artery aneurysm, and 1 patient was treated by removal of a foreign body in the common femoral artery. 2 patients required an operation after developing large hematoma.

It is important to consider the relatively low cost of a PTA compared to an arterial bypass procedure. However, many of the patients required an additional surgical intervention and therefore the total cost was higher than that of an uncomplicated bypass.

38 patients required only one operation, after the ill-fated PTA, whereas 9 required two interventious. 2 required three further interventions, 1 patient four operations, another five and the limit being reached by two patients requiring six and 11 reinterventions respectively.

The surgical complications which required further hospitalisation can be analyzed as follows:

Bypass occlusion in 6 cases, below-knee amputation in 1 case, above-knee amputation in 4 cases, a post-operative embolus in the treated leg in 1 case, hematoma development in 4 patients, development of a paralytic ileus and pulmonary edema in one patient, a lesion of the femoral nerve in 2 patients and infection of the surgical wound in another 2 patients. The worst complication of patient death during angioplasty or as result of a failed PTA attempt is only mentioned rarely in the literature. This tragic, fortunately rare outcome, we experienced in 3 patients at our hospital.

Discussion

In conclusion, it can be said that PTA is a frequently used procedure for the early treatment of peripheral vascular disease which has markedly increased our therapeutic options. However, after having taken a closer look at the possible complications after a PTA attempt some arguments promoting a PTA rather than vascular reconstructions in selected cases are no longer viable. This has been frequently pointed out by vascular surgeons. First of all, one should adhere to strict indications when promoting a PTA attempt.

Secondly, a close monitoring of the patient during and after the angioplasty is to be closely adhered to, since it has been proven that early intervention using vascular surgical possibilities has frequently led to better results for the patient. Even when keeping in mind the possible complications of a PTA when using this technique for chronic peripheral vascular disease, the use of a PTA prior to vascular reconstruction can be promoted.

This requires close interaction between radiologists and surgeons in the setting of indications. One should also never allow the patient to choose which type of therapy appeals to him, and he should be adequately being informed of the risks of both procedures.

Author's address:
Simone Ricke, MD
Chirurgische Klinik
Akademisches Lehrkrankenhaus Porz
Universität zu Köln
Urbacher Weg 19
51149 Köln, Germany

Iliofemoral versus axillofemoral bypass for unilateral inflow reconstruction

D. Arvanitis

Department of Vascular Surgery, Athens General Hospital, Athens, Greece

Aortobifemoral bypass is the treatment of choice for symptomatic aortoiliac arterial occlusive disease (1). However in high-risk patients, this procedure is related with a considerable morbidity and mortality (8). For these patients and for those with unilateral iliac disease many other alternatives have been proposed, having lower rate of operative morbidity and mortality. These procedures include the iliac endarterectomies, the miscellaneous endovascular procedures, the various extraanatomical and the iliofemoral bypasses (2, 7). All these previous types of repair avoid intraabdominal surgery. Endarterectomies have limited indications, with the best results reported in the cases where the disease is localized to the infrarenal aorta and the common iliac vessels (1, 9). Endovascular surgery is indicated in short segments and mainly in non obstructing lesions and needs highly equipped institutions. For most Vascular Units extraanatomical and iliofemoral bypasses remain the routine way of repair for obstructing unilateral iliac lesions. The aim of the present study is to analyze and compare the outcome of 42 unilateral iliofemoral and 35 axillounifemoral bypasses, performed during an 8-year period on high risk patients with unilateral iliac or iliofemoral disease and severe leg ischemia.

Patients and methods

In an 8-year period (1986 − 1994) 77 patients underwent unilateral iliofemoral (n = 42) or axillofemoral (n = 35) bypass. There were 68 males and 9 females. The mean age of the iliofemoral group was 65.8 years (SD = 9.6 range 44 − 88) and of the axillofemoral group 73.5 years (SD = 6.7 range 62 − 86). The indication for inflow reconstruction in the iliofemoral group was severe intermittent claudication in 4. rest pain in 25 and gangrene toes in 13 patients. The corresponding indications for the axillounifemoral group were severe intermittent claudication in 1, rest pain in 18, and peripheral gangrene in 16 patients. The only criterion to perform a unilateral iliofemoral bypass was a patent ipsilateral common iliac artery. The criterion to perform a unilateral axillofemoral bypass was the absence of a patent segment of the common iliac artery in high-risk patients (ASA III−IV) not amenable for aortic surgery. All iliofemoral procedures were performed with the standard retroperitoneal approach. All the iliofemoral were elective cases, however 8 axillofemoral bypasses (23 %) were performed as emergency procedures. As a routine, iliofemoral bypass was performed under spinal anesthesia. In selective cases general anesthesia was employed.

Results

The 1-year, 2-year and 5-year secondary cumulative patency rate for the iliofemoral group was 92.5 %, 90 % and 86.5 % (life table method). The corresponding patency rates for the axillofemoral group were 87.8 %, 83 % and 60 %.

The operative mortality for both groups (defined as death within 30 postoperative days) was 5 % (2/42) and 6 % (2/35). Five iliofemoral (12 %) and 7 axillofemoral bypasses (20 %) thrombosed during the follow-up period. However, non-thrombotic complications occurred in the axillofemoral group (four infected grafts, two of them after a perigraft seroma formation, one false aneurysm in the proximal axillary anastomosis and one case with arterial steal and arm ischemia.

Conclusions

1. Iliofemoral bypass is the operation of choice for unilateral iliac obstruction in cases with a patent segment of the common iliac artery. Long-term results of this procedure are competitive to that of the standard aortofemoral grafts with patency rates well over 90 % at 3-years (2, 4, 6).
2. Axillounifemoral bypasses are inferior to the iliofemoral ones not only because of the lower patency rate ranging at 5-years (3, 5) but for a considerable rate of other complications such as infection, false aneurysm formation etc. The only indication for unilateral axillofemoral bypass is the inability to insert an iliofemoral graft in high-risk patients.

References

1. Brewster DC, Darling RC (1978) Optimal methods of aortoiliac reconstructions. Surgery 84: 739–
2. Couch NP, Clowes AW, Whitemore AD, Lombara JA, Henderson BA, Mannick JA (1985) The iliac origin arterial graft: a useful alternative for iliac occlusive disease. Surg 97: 83–87
3. Eugene J, Goldstone J, Moore WS (1977) Fifteen-year experience with subcutaneous bypass grafts for lower extremely ischemia. Ann Surg 186: 177–183
4. Kallman PG, Hosang M, Johnston KW, Walter PM (1987) Unilateral iliac disease. J Vasc Surg 6: 139–143
5. LoGerfo FW, Johnson WC, Corson JD et al. (1977) A comparison of the late patency rates of axillobilateral femoral and axillounilateral femoral grafts. Surg 81: 33–40
6. Perler BA, Burdick JF, Williams GM (1991) Femorofemoral or iliofemoral bypass for unilateral inflow reconstruction. Am J Surg 161: 426–430
7. Rutherford RB, Patt A, Pearce WH (1987) Extraanatomic bypass: a closer view. J Vasc Surg 6: 437–446
8. Schaeffer D, Koepf R et al. (1982) Operatives Vorgehen bei Rekonstruktionen der Aortenbifurkation. Angio Archiv 3
9. Szillagyi DE, Smith RF, Whitney DG (1964) The durability of aortoiliac endarterectomy. Arch Surg 89

Author's address:
Dimitrios Arvanitis, MD
Department of Vascular Surgery
Athens General Hospital
154 Mesogion Ave
11527 Athens, Greece

Femoro-popliteal bypass: indication, material choice, technique, results

P. Apostolidis

"Asklipio" General Hospital of Voula, Athens, Greece

Non-operative procedures have become a popular alternative to peripheral bypass surgery in selected patients with peripheral vascular disease of the lower extremities, but are really indicated in the treatment of claudication; rarely the percutaneous angioplastic techniques are indicated in the end stage limb ischemia where leg bypass procedures are in order for limb salvage. In fact, combination of both types of treatment sometimes is necessary.

It is important to bear in mind that frequently the blood flow to the lower limbs is restored automatically and to look for the occasion when this may take place merely with the passage of time to provide an excellent clinical result without performing any intervention.

Indication

Almost all of the patients considered for this type of reconstruction have atherosclerosis. Most of the patients are male and usually between the ages 40 – 75. Nearly every patient has smoked more than 20 cigarettes per day for 20 years or more. Approximately 30 % of the patients will have had a myocardial infarction or severe coronary disease and more than 45 % are diabetic. In most patients the indication for grafting and bypassing the femoral and popliteal artery is critical ischemia, threatened limb loss and severe disabling intermittent claudication.

So, in patients whose limbs are threatened because of infrainguinal arteriosclerosis, femoro-distal reconstruction should be considered and attempted if feasible, unless gangrene extends into the deeper tissues of the tarsal region of the foot or unless the patient has severe organic mental syndrome with inability to ambulate, communicate or provide self-care. Patients in the later category or those with severe long-standing flexion contractures should undergo primary above- or below-knee amputations. Unusual indications for femoro-distal reconstruction are failed angioplastic procedures in acute or sub-acute cases thomboses of femoral or popliteal arteries that thrombectomy is not successful, thrombosis of popliteal aneurysm and occasionally traumatic lesions (even iatrogenic) of the thigh and knee arteries.

When indicated, it is worthwhile to attempt some type of reconstruction for lowering the amputation level: at any age, a below-knee amputation is much more preferable than the above-knee.

Material choice

The saphenous vein, preferably reversed, – or in situ – remains the material of choice for the infrainguinal arterial bypass procedures with the distal anastomoses either above or below the knee, and there is no point in preserving this vein for possible cardiac or other procedures.

The second choice, should the saphenous or even the cephalic vein be small or unusable, is a PTFE graft either alone or in a composite fashion, using some kind of vein in the distal part of the bypass. Of course, in patients with life expectancy of less then 3 years, and for above-knee procedures, the decision to use synthetic grafts is easier.

The strengthened with Dacron mesh umbilical veins are the next best choice and similar results with PTFE grafts should be expected although this has to be documented.

Other materials have unacceptable results and should be avoided. Sequential – "jump" – bypass, or bypass to an isolated segment to popliteal artery (more then 7 cm in length) using even different materials, and several other methods, mainly in the performance of the distal anastomosis, are reported to give good results that are not always reproducible by others.

Results

In the last 20 years the primary amputation rate fell from 45 % to 14 % ; this is due to better understanding of the hemodynamics, the advent of the different techniques of non-operative techniques and the better materials used, along with improved techniques.

For above-knee bypass, in the first 2 years, the results are similar when comparing autologous veins to synthetic material-PTFE-70 % to 80 % patency rate, but is clearly favorable to the autologous material in the fourth year-65 % for the veins and 40 % – 45 % for the PTFE, the difference increasing more in the 5th year.

In the distal to the knee bypass procedures, where the 1-year patency rate is similar-70 % to 75 %, there is a real difference from the second to the 5th year: 60 % to 35 %, that increases as the time passes. The composite grafts are somewhere between these results.

The 30-day mortality rate for these operations is between 5 % and 10 %.

From all these patients submitted to limb salvage operations, more than 50 % are expected to die in the first 5 years, but for those that remain alive more than 75 % will keep walking.

Nevertheless, because of the excellent palliation achieved by this active operative approach to limb salvage, in most patients it seems worthwhile to make an effort to save that limb.

Author's address:
Petros Apostolidis, MD
"Asklipio" General Hospital of Voula
1, Vas. Pavlou str.,
16673 Voula, Athens, Greece

Femoro-distal PTFE bypass reconstruction with vein collar

M. Lazarides

Department of Vascular Surgery, Athens General Hospital, Athens, Greece

In patients requiring femorodistal bypasses, autologous vein conduits remain the graft of choice for revascularization of a threatened limb. Saphenous vein either in situ or reversed, arm veins and composite vein grafts have been used. However in a small number of patients especially in secondary and tertiary reconstructions the use of a non-vein prosthetic alternative may be required. PTFE graft is the routine for most vascular surgeons when autologous vein is not available. Unfortunately, long-term patency rates of femorodistal PTFE grafts are disappointing and range from 7 % to 22 % at 3 years (6, 11).

We have attempted to improve these disappointing results by fashioning a venous cuff at the distal anastomosis using additional routine long-term anticoagulation and we report our results with 17 consecutive femorodistal PTFE grafts.

Patients and methods

In a 4-year period 17 PTFE femorodistal arterial reconstructions with venous cuff technique were performed in 16 patients. Their age ranged from 46 to 90 years (mean 71.6), 6 were men and 10 women. The distal anastomosis was performed in the anterior tibial artery in 10 limbs, in the posterior tibial in 6 and in the peroneal artery in one. Indication for surgery was rest pain in 8 and peripheral gangrene in 9 limbs. Four were secondary and 3 tertiary reconstructions. All patients received long-term oral anticoagulation (acenocoumarol).

Results

Follow-up ranged 7 to 58 months (mean 20 months). Eight grafts occluded during that period and the cumulative 1-year and 2-year patency rate was 70 % and 54 % respectively. Four patients underwent major amputations and the cumulative limb salvage rate was calculated 75 % at 2 years. The operative mortality was zero, however one patient was complicated with upper gastrointestinal bleeding necessitating temporary discontinuance of the anticoagulants.

Discussion

The venous cuff technique was first reported from Siegman (7) and was modified by Miller (4) to facilitate the anastomosis of rigid grafts to small arteries. The theoretical advantages of a venous cuff at the distal anastomosis include 1) easier and more accurate completion of the anastomosis and avoidance of distortion, which may improve the initial patency rate and 2) less myointimal hyperplasia accumulation, which may improve the long-term patency rate. Reduction of myointimal hyperplasia accumulation is achieved by the interposition of a more compliant conduit between the compliant artery and the less compliant rigid prosthesis, as compliance mismatching is a well known cause of myointimal hyperplasia development. The longitudinal compliance of a vein is greater than the transverse compliance and subsequently the venous cuff is more compliant than the normally orientated vein in a conventional composite graft (8, 9).

In a review of the literature only three articles were found reporting cumulative patency rates of femorodistal PTFE bypasses with venous cuff, ranging 51 % – 62 % at 1-year and 29 – 62 % at 2-years (2, 5, 10). Our competitive results with 70 % patency at 1-year may reflect the influence of the long-term oral anticoagulation which has not been stretched in the previous reports. Postoperative oral anticoagulation treatment has received little attention despite some reported encouraging results (1, 3). In conclusion, our limited experience in femorodistal PTFE bypasses using venous cuff and long-term oral anticoagulation strongly supports its use for reconstructions to the infrapopliteal level in limbs which lack sufficient autologous veins.

References

1. Flinn WR, Rohrer MJ, Yao JST et al. (1988) Improved long-term patency of infragenicular PTFE grafts. J Vasc Surg 7: 685–690
2. Harris PL, Bakran A, Enabi L, Nott DM (1993) ePTFE grafts for femorocrural by-pass, improved results with combined adjuvant venous cuff and arteriovenous fistula? Eur J Vasc Surg 7: 528–533
3. Kretschmer G, Herbst F, Prager M et al. (1992) A decade of oral anticoagulant treatment to maintain autologous vein grafts for femoropopliteal atherosclerosis. Arch Surg 127: 1112–1115
4. Miller JH, Foreman RK, Ferguson L, Faris I (1984) Interposition vein cuff for anastomosis of prosthesis to small artery. Aust NZ J Surg 54: 283–285
5. Morris GE, Raptis S, Miller JH, Faris IB (1993) Femorocrural grafting and regrafting: does PTFE have a role? Eur J Vasc Surg 7: 3290–334
6. Quinones-Baldrich WJ, Prego AA, Ucelay-Gomez R et al. (1992) Long term results of infrainguinal revascularization with PTFE, a ten-year experience. J Vasc Surg 16: 209–217
7. Siegman FA (1979) Use of the venous cuff for graft anastomosis. Surg Gynec Obstet 148: 930–
8. Suggs WD, Henriques HF, DePalma RG (1988) Vein cuff interposition prevents juxta-anastomotic neo-intimal hyperplasia. Ann Surg 207: 717–723
9. Tyrrell MR, Chester JF, Vipond MN, Clarke GH, Taylor RS, Wolfe JHN (1990) Experimental evidence to support the use of interposition vein collars/patches in distal PTFE anastomoses. Eur J Vasc Surg 4: 95–101
10. Wolfe JHN, Tyrrell MR (1991) Justifying arterial reconstruction to crural vessels even with a prosthetic graft. Br J Surg 78: 897–899
11. Yeager RA, Hobson RW, Hamil Z, Lynch TG, Lee BC, Jain K (1982) Differential patency and limb salvage for PTFE and saphenous vein in severe lower extremity ischemia. Surgery 91: 99–103

Author's address:
Miltos Lazarides, MD
Department of Vascular Surgery
Athens General Hospital
154 Mesogion Ave
11527 Athens, Greece

Appendix

Four additional patients were operated using the vein cuff technique since the last presentation of the preliminary data 20 months ago. There were two men and two women and the distal anastomosis was performed in the anterior tibial in two and in the posterior tibial artery in two cases. The cumulative patency rate after a mean follow-up of 24 months and the new cases added was 54 % and 48 % in 1 and 2 years respectively (Kaplan-Meier method). Although there was an expected drop in the 1-year patency rate this is still quite acceptable in cases where there is no autologous vein available.

Crural and pedal bypass surgery: surgical technique and results

H. Schweiger

Herz- und Gefäßklinik, Rhön-Klinikum, Bad Neustadt, Germany

In all civilized countries there is an increasing number of patients suffering from diabetes for 10 or 20 years or even longer. About 50 % of all patients presenting with limb threatening ischemia are diabetics. In most of these cases, peripheral arterial occlusive disease (POD) is located below the inguinal ligament, and often in the lower leg arteries exclusively. Clinical examination shows a palpable popliteal pulse but absent ankle pulses. The typical angiographic pattern is a total occlusion of all three lower leg vessels with the popliteal or superficial femoral artery patent. Almost always, some kind of a plantar arch or parts of it are present. Since most of these patients are facing lower leg amputation the question arises, whether vein bypass surgery to the plantar arch can preserve the leg despite this limited outflow tract.

Materials and methods

A series of 37 short pedal vein grafts was performed in 34 patients. The mean age of the patients was 72 years and 30 % were female, 92 % had diabetes and the mean duration of diabetes was 18 years. Although one-third of the cases had impaired renal function, none of them was on dialysis. Clinical examination revealed a positive popliteal pulse, but negative ankle pulses. Angiography showed in all cases a complete occlusion of all three lower leg vessels and, mostly, some kind of a plantar arch. Every patient with this pattern of POD was considered to be a candidate for reconstruction, except there was no Doppler signal on the pedal or posterior tibial artery below the ankle.

Thirty-six legs showed necrosis or gangrene and one rest pain. Minor amputation had been performed in nearly one-third of the patients which did not heal. The greater saphenous vein was used as graft material in all cases, either reversed or non-reversed after cutting the valves. The proximal anastomosis was performed always with the popliteal artery above (8 cases) or below the knee (29 cases). The distal anastomosis was performed with the pedal artery (14), the posterior tibial artery at or below the ankle (21 cases), or both (two cases).

After completion of the distal anastomosis, peripheral resistance was measured, as described previously (1). Long-term anticoagulation was never used in these patients. Complete follow-up could be obtained in all cases. The sole parameter for graft function was a palpable bypass graft at the site of the distal anastomosis.

Results

No patient died within the first 30 days after the operation. Ten graft failures occurred during the first 2 months resulting in lower leg amputation in seven patients. Two further graft failures were seen, 3 months and 7 months after the operation, respectively. In these two cases the limb could be saved since the peripheral lesions had been healed. The cumulative (secondary) bypass graft patency rate was 78 % after 1 month, 69 % after 6 months, and 66 % after 60 months. Beyond the first year no graft failure was observed.

There were some factors which influenced graft patency. The 1 month patency rate was 90 % when the vein was of good quality and > 4 mm in size. In contrast, veins with a diameter ≤ 4 mm showed a 67 % patency rate after this time. Another factor was the status of the plantar arch. However, the differences in patency in patients having a complete arch versus an incomplete arch was not significant. Resistance measurements, however, where a good indicator for early graft failure. When the resistance value was 1500 mPRU or more (six cases) no graft remained patent.

The limb salvage rate was 77 % after 9 months and remained constant up to 5 years. In the early period after the operation, one patient had to be amputated despite a functioning graft. After the minor amputation had healed, a heel necrosis occurred necessitating amputation. In addition, another patient was amputated > 5 years after the operation due to chronic osteomyelitis with a functioning graft.

Discussion

The present results indicate that short pedal vein grafts show an excellent patency in limbs with isolated occlusion below the popliteal level. It is well known that short vein grafts to the pedal arteries have a better prognosis compared to long femoro-distal vein bypasses (2–4). Since the number of diabetic patients is increasing, it is assumed that patients with isolated lower leg POD will also be seen more frequently. A successful revascularisation in patients with palpable popliteal pulse but absent ankle pulses can control peripheral gangrene and allow heeling following minor amputation.

References

1. Schweiger H, Lang W (1992) Klinische Bedeutung des peripheren Gefäßwiderstandes für die frühe Bypassverschlußrate – Fehler und Gefahren bei der Widerstandsmessung. Vasa (Suppl) 36: 14–17
2. Veith FJ et al. (1985) Tibiotibial vein bypass-grafts: a new operation for limb salvage. J Vasc Surg 2: 552
3. Wölfle KD et al. (1987) Distale Bypassoperationen bei peripherer arterieller Verschlußkrankheit: eine Alternative zur primären Amputation? Angio 9: 345
4. Schweiger H, Lang W (1992) Die diabetische Gangrän bei peripheren Gefäßverschlüssen. Chirurg 63: 438

Author's address:
Prof. Dr. H. Schweiger
Herz- und Gefäßklinik
Rhön-Klinikum
97616 Bad Neustadt, Germany

Intra-operative measurements: The role of peripheral resistance

H. Bruijnen, K. D. Woelfle, C. Fitz, H. Loeprecht

Department of Thoracic and Vascular Surgery, Zentralklinikum Augsburg, Germany

Introduction

Many questions have been raised which factors play a role in early occlusion of infra-inguinal bypasses. To answer the question, whether the peripheral resistance plays a role in this matter, we have investigated 54 consecutive patients, who received a femoropopliteal or femorodistal bypass at our institution during the first half year of 1994. The bypass material was saphenous vein in most cases, or ePTFE: (Gore Tex®) or composed of these two materials (composite bypass).

As one can see from the above sketch fluid is instilled into the proximal end of the bypass before completion of the proximal anastomosis. A thin cannula for pressure measurement is put into the bypass at the level of the distal anastomosis. Before the fluid instillation is started, the bypass is clamped slightly proximal of the lower anastomosis and the prevailing pressure is recorded – collateral back pressure (CBP). After this measurement the fluid application into the bypass is started at increasing quantities: 25, 50, 100 and 150 ml/min. The corresponding systolic, mean and diastolic pressures are measured by a transducer and printed out on paper for documentation. These measurements are repeated after application of a vasodilatatory drug, in our series papaverin. The OR is calculated by

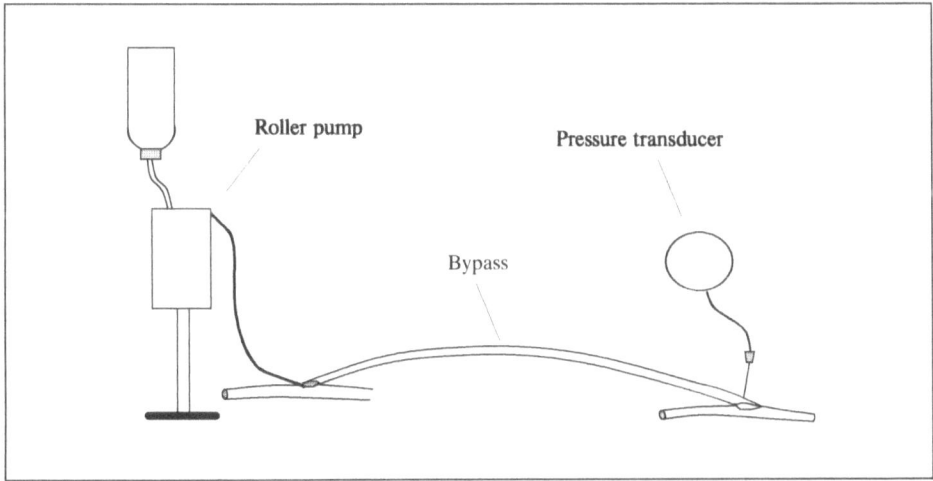

Fig. 1. Description of the measurement method for the determination of the peripheral arterial resistance (OR).

dividing the prevailing pressure by the applied fluid quantity. The value is expressed as peripheral resistance units (PRU), after division by 1000 as mPRU.

Apart from measuring these OR and CBP values before releasing blood flow, we also measure blood flow and the prevailing pressure at the lower end of the bypass. Dividing this pressure by flow results into a somewhat more physiological value, which we have called completion resistance (COR). This value sometimes is cited in the literature as impedance at zero frequency. We have calculated a flowindex by dividing flow by pressure (formula shown below). Apart from these values other bypass related factors were used as prognostic variables for multivariate analysis to investigate, whether one can predict bypass occlusion within 30 days. These factors are listed in the following table:

Table 1. Studies variables

Dependent variable:
    Bypass occlusion < 30 days

Independent nominal variables:
    Distal anastomosis
    Monbypass y/n
    Bypassmaterial
    revision because of angiography
    revision because of angioscopy

Independent quantitative variables:
    resistance
    resistance after vasodilatation
    collateral back pressure
    CBP after vasodilatation
    flowindex
    vein length
    ePTFE length
    total length

Measurement methods

The resistance is calculated without and with vasodilatation by papaverin according to the formula:

$$R = \frac{\text{measured mean pressure}}{\text{mean flow}}$$

After restoring the blood flow the flow index can be calculated according to the formula:

$$\text{Flowindex} = \frac{\text{measured mean flow}}{\text{measured mean pressure}}$$

Statistical analysis

Our analysis was performed in following steps. Firstly the so-called point-biserial correlation of all independent variables with the dependent variable (bypass occlusion < 30 days y/n) is calculated. The result is shown in table 2. The corresponding bar graph is shown in figure 2.

Table 2. Correlation

	r	significance (%)
resistance	-0.0119	7.03
resistance after vasodil.	-0.0153	8.89
collat. Backpressure	-0.0312	17.59
CBP after vasodil.	-0.0638	35.35
flowindex	-0.1217	61.95
distal anastomosis	0.4847	58.99
monobypass y/n	-0.3162	98.01
vein/ePTFE	-0.1039	51.83
diameter	-0.1390	68.38
bypass length	0.4378	99.90
revision because of angiography	0.4667	99.96
revision because of angioscopy	0.3730	99.47

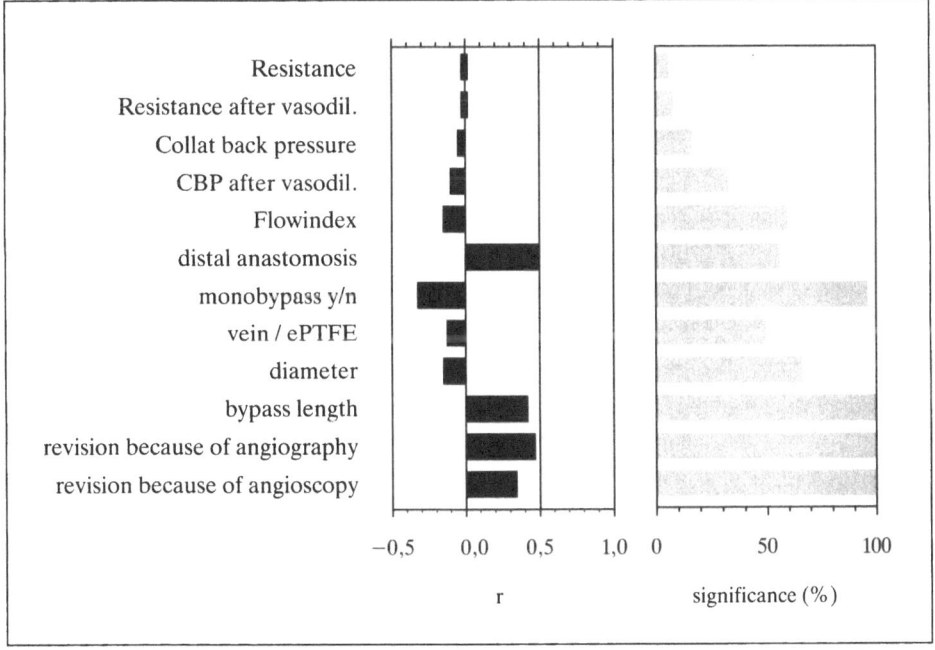

Fig. 2. Correlation with occlusion

After this preliminary step of correlation calculation, the main procedure of the statistical analysis – multiple logistic regression analysis – is started. With this method of statistical evaluation one tries to find out, which independent variables predict the outcome of the dependent variable best. The logistic transformation is done, while the dependent variable is nominal with two values (yes, no). With logistic transformation one gets the probabilities, that the event will occur for the various combinations of the independent variables. We have performed a stepwise backward analysis, where the insignificant variables are eliminated after each step, creating several models with a decreasing number of independent, sometimes called predictor variables. Our first model was calculated with all independent variables (model 1). The total variability should be seen as the spreading of the individual observation, the explained variability as the part, which can be explained by the calculated model. The significance is calculated with the variance ratio test (F-test) and should be over 95 % (corresponds with $p < 0.05$). The result is shown in table 3.

The significance of the model as a whole is expressed by the quantity R^2, which is calculated by the following formula:

$$R^2 = \frac{\text{explained variability}}{\text{total variability}}$$

For our model 1 this quantity is 0.9999, which is not astonishing, while all independent variables were included. This kind of model cannot be useful in daily surgical practice, because it includes all variables.

In the following you will see the results of the models we have calculated together with some comments. The results are listed in tables like the previous table 3 and mostly self explaining. Due to technical reasons the multiple logistic regression analysis after removing the insignificant variables CBP, vein length, distal anastomosis, revision related to the angioscopic from model leads to a so-called saturated model, which could not be

Table 3. Multiple logistic analysis with all independent variables

	Variability	significance (F-test)
total	212.5876	
explained	212.5649	96.55
resistance	3.9980	95.31
resistance after vasodil.	3.7251	96.13
CBP	2.9735	94.51
CBP after vasodil.	3.6713	95.09
Flowindex	4.3046	95.49
Diameter	11.0013	97.18
vein length	0.6722	87.90
ePTFE length	13.0982	97.40
distal anastomosis	30.7078	94.78
bypass material	10.5329	97.12
revision rel. to angiography	30.1889	98.18
revision rel. to angioscopy	2.2156	93.57

evaluated. Therefore we had to give up the logistic transformation of the dependent variable. Model 2 is then calculated without logistic transformation.

Table 4. Results of model 2

	Variability	Significance (%)
total	7.0833	
explained	1.8301	94.10
Resistance	0.0687	54.29
Resistance after vasodil.	0.0089	20.95
CBP after vasodil.	0.0011	7.63
flowindex	0.0501	47.54
bypass material	0.0293	37.34
revision rel. to angiography	1.3801	99.83

$$R^2 = 0.2584.$$

The explanatory power of this model is very low, although it is nearly significant with 94.10 %.

After this disappointing result we tried an analysis with the hemodynamic parameters (model 3), with the following results.

Table 5. Analysis with hemodynamic parameters

	Variability	Significance (%)
total	7.5000	
explained	0.2182	8.31
resistance	0.0050	14.27
resistance after vasodil.	0.0001	1.55
CBP	0.0043	13.35
CBP after vasodil.	0.0264	32.20
flowindex	0.1729	70.90

$$R^2 = 0.0291.$$

This means that the hemodynamic parameters alone explain almost nothing concerning the occurence of a bypass occlusion within the first 30 days after operation.

Next analysis step: multiple regression with all quantitative parameters (model 4).

Table 6. Analysis with all quantitative parameters

	Variability	Significance (%)
	7.5000	
explained	2.5074	98.74
resistance	0.0291	38.97
resistance after vasodil.	0.0232	35.10
CBP	0.1226	70.14
CBP after vasodil.	0.2652	87.07
flowindex	0.4141	94.04
diameter	0.1382	72.97
vein length	1.7522	99.98
ePTFE length	1.8225	99.99

$$R^2 = 0.3343,$$

meaning this model explains about one 1/3 of the variability.

For the calculation of the next model (model 5) the totally insignificant resistance variables are excluded, vein length and ePTFE length are taken together as total length. The results are shown in table 7.

Table 7. Analysis with the significant quantitative parameters (model 5)

	Variability	Significance (%)
total	7.5000	
explained	2.4456	99.81
CBP	0.0735	59.25
CBP after vasodil.	0.2334	85.68
flowindex	0.4508	95.61
diameter	0.4375	95.30
total length	2.0826	100.00

$$R^2 = 0.3261.$$

Herewith this model also is not performing well in predicting the outcome of the dependent variable – bypass occlusion < 30 days –, although the significance of the explained variability is 99.81 %.

For the model 6 the insignificant collateral back pressure variables are eliminated. The results are displayed in table 8.

Table 8. Results of model 6

	Variability	Significance (%)
total	7.5000	
explained	2.1625	99.91
flowindex	0.3596	92.76
diameter	0.3707	93.18
total length	1.9140	100.00

$$R^2 = 0.2883.$$

The model explains very little of the total variability occurring in reality, although again significant with 99.91 %. Secondly the bypass length seems to be the only significant quantitative variable.

In the next model 7 we combined the significant nominal and quantitative variables from the previous models. For the results see table 9.

Table 9. Analysis with the significant nominal and quantitative variables

	Variability	Significance (%)
total	7.5000	
explained	2.7955	99.99
revision rel. to angiography	1.3581	99.97
total length	1.1621	99.91

$$R^2 = 0.3727.$$

Although this model is highly significant, it explains very little, as shown by the quantity R^2.

Because the dependent variable is a yes/no nominal variable, we have performed the analysis again after logistic transformation, giving the possibility of calculating probabilities of the event occlusion within 30 days for various subgroups (model 8). Table 10 is showing the results.

Table 10. Logistic regression analysis with significant nominal and quantitative variables

	Variability	Significance (%)
total	467.3446	
explained	246.7783	99.99
revision rel. to angiography	125.5733	99.99
total length	71.8503	99.66

$$R^2 = 0.528.$$

Although the model is highly significant with 99.99 %, corresponding to p < 0.0001, the explanatory power is poor.

Table 11 shows the results of the analysis of the observed and expected frequencies, that the bypass will remain patent during the first 30 days postop. There are differences up to almost 40 %. It seems that this, our best, model cannot be applied to predict the outcome of infra-inguinal bypasses.

Table 11. Analysis of observed and expected frequencies (model 8)

Revision	Length	expected	observed	difference
no	20–30	0.999	1.00	−0.001
no	30–40	0.996	1.00	−0.004
no	40–50	0.984	0.89	−0.095
no	50–60	0.938	1.00	−0.062
no	60–70	0.792	1.00	−0.208
yes	20–30	0.863	1.00	−0.137
yes	30–40	0.613	1.00	−0.387
yes	40–50	0.285	0.00	0.285
yes	50–60	0.091	0.00	0.091
yes	60–70	0.025	0.00	0.025

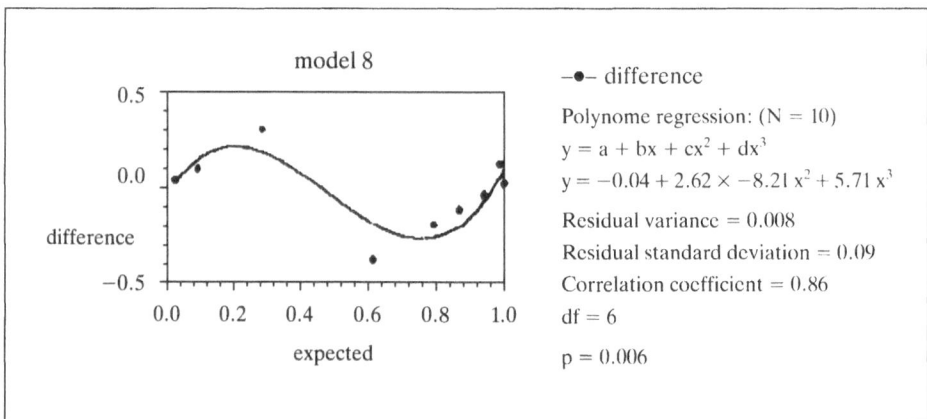

model 8

−●– difference

Polynome regression: (N = 10)

$y = a + bx + cx^2 + dx^3$

$y = -0.04 + 2.62 \times -8.21\,x^2 + 5.71\,x^3$

Residual variance = 0.008

Residual standard deviation = 0.09

Correlation coefficient = 0.86

df = 6

p = 0.006

Fig. 3. Analysis of observed and expected frequencies

In good models, the differences should be in the same range around zero for all expected frequencies. As is shown in the graph, there is rather a cubic relationship between the observed and expected frequencies. It is clear, that such a model with this kind of relation between the observed and expected frequencies cannot be used in clinical medicine for predicting outcomes.

Table 12. Goodness-of-fit and significance of all models

Model	Goodness-of-fit	Significance
1	0.9999	96.55
2	0.2584	94.10
3	0.0291	8.31
4	0.3343	98.74
5	0.3261	99.81
6	0.2883	99.91
7	0.3727	99.99
8	0.528	99.99

Conclusions

– Resistance does not play a role in predicting graft occlusion < 30 days.
– Bypass length and angiography related revision seem to be more important.
– The "goodness-of-fit" is bad in all models, as is shown in the final table 12.
– There is more "on this earth" to explain or predict bypass occlusion than we can measure in every day clinical practice.

Author's address:
Hans Bruijnen
Dept. of Vascular and Thoracic Surgery
Zentralklinikum Augsburg
Stenglinstrasse 2
86156 Augsburg, Germany

Spinal cord stimulation in non-reconstructable or daredevil reconstructable patients with critical limb ischemia

L. Claeys, K. Ktenidis, S. Horsch

Department of General and Vascular Surgery, Krankenhaus Porz am Rhein, Academic Teaching Hospital of the University of Cologne, Germany

Spinal cord stimulation for chronic pain

The Gate Theory of pain transmission in the dorsal horn of the spinal cord provided the foundation for the use of electrical stimulation for pain relief.

After initial promising results, use of electrical stimulation became widespread, but poor understanding of patient selection criteria yielded disappointing outcome in many cases.

Spinal cord stimulation for chronic ischemic pain

Albert W. Cook (1973), a neurosurgeon from New York, was the first to try spinal cord stimulation in patients with peripheral vascular disease.

Ten years later, different workers presented data showing significant pain relief and ulcer healing in non-reconstructable patients under SCS.

Selection of the vascular patient for stimulation therapy

The fate of the patient suffering from critical limb ischemia is poor. The first treatment options to consider are endovascular procedures and vascular reconstructions.

For distal bypass, the failure rate is at least 30 % within the first year. Once a vein graft occludes the results of desobliteration and revision are dismal, with 5-year patencies ranging from 5 to 32 %. Redo surgery is difficult and often impossible when there are no suitable recipient arteries or when the supply of veins has been exhausted. If prosthetic grafts are used, long-term patency rates are even poorer.

But, when is a patient non-reconstructable or inoperable? It is evident that inoperability should have a number of definitions and that this definition is accepted among the vascular surgeons.

However, it is impossible to expect full conformity with a definition, but we should aim for all studies presenting new treatments to include the same criteria in order to compare and interpret data. Then we will be able to find predictors of clinical outcome.

In our opinion, we should distinguish between the primary and secondary non-reconstructable patient:

- Primary non-reconstructability or the inoperable patient before any attempt at revascularization

  Reasons for rejecting attempts at revascularization are: reconstruction inappropriate, unsafe, impossible or inadvisable:

  - necrosis of a major part of the limb
  - life-threatening toxemia
  - no operable distal vessels
  - reconstruction technically possible, but with poor chance of success

- Secondary non-reconstructability or the inoperable patient after an attempt at revascularization

  - no operable distal vessels
  - vein not available

- Other reasons for inoperability are no informed consent available or general inoperability.

But how to define the technically reconstructable patient "with poor chance of long-term success".

Should we force distal or pedal bypass surgery, carrying the risk that early failure results in an amputation at a higher level than would have been necessary. And if repeated re-exploration was able to save the bypass, have we also saved a useful functional limb?

And how to manage graft occlusion and recurrent limb ischemia? Different options are available such as surgical thrombectomy with or without a secondary procedures, thrombolysis of the graft and catheter-based techniques.

Treatment modalities for non-reconstructable patients

Pharmacotherapy: Different studies have reported beneficial effects of prostaglandins on ischemic pain and ulcer healing in non-reconstructable patients.

Sympathectomy: Because of doubts about its efficacy, the number of surgical sympathectomies has decreased during the last two decades. It is sometimes used as a last resort in non-reconstructable patients with intractable pain conditions or superficial skin ulcers, and in patients with thromboangiitis obliterans.

Spinal cord stimulation: Spinal cord stimulation relieves ischemic pain and increases skin blood flow. Effects on limb salvage remains to be examined.

Mechanisms of action of spinal cord stimulation

Electrical stimulation of the spinal cord for ischemic pain, and as last resort in ischemic conditions, can develop into an important tool in the management of non-reconstructable

limb ischemia. Despite the clinical value of the method, the knowledge of the mechanisms underlying the resulting effects has been scanty. At present, the mechanisms proposed to be responsible for the modulation of ischemic pain are neurophysiological and neurochemical in nature:
– direct inhibition of nociceptive transmission in the spinothalamic tracts
– antidromic activation of high threshold afferents
– local release of vasoactive substances
– depression of sympathetically maintained vasoconstrictor activity.

Questions to be examined

– Is SCS effective for the relief of ischemic pain?
– Does SCS promotes ulcer healing?
– Is there a limb-saving effect?
– Is SCS cost effective?
– What are the complications?
– How does it works?

Results of SCS in limb ischemia: A review of published data

– Pain relief:	about 70 % success
– Ulcer healing:	about 50 % success
– Limb survival:	about 65 – 70 % success
– Complications:	technical: 10 %
	surgical: < 5 %

German experience with SCS for critical limb ischemia n = 408

	Stage III	Stage IV
Cologne: (Horsch et al.)	169	68
Nuremberg: (Raithel et al.)	88	53
Munich: (Lauterjung et al.)	18	12
Total	275	133

	Pain relief	Ulcer healing	Limb survival	Follow-up
C:	72 %	45 %	68 %	48 m.
N:	65 %	35 %	78 %	36 m.
M:	83 %	40 %	74 %	± ly.

Cologne-randomized study "SCS+PGE1" vs. "PGE1"

Patients and methods

A randomized controlled study was made of 86 patients with Fontaine stage IV (CLI) undergoing intravenous prostaglandin therapy for nonhealing ischemic foot ulcers.

All patients had arteriosclerosis, and 13 had diabetes mellitus.

Entry criteria included: CLI with ankle systolic pressure less than 50 mm Hg, foot trans-cutaneous oxygen $TcPO_2$ less than 20 mm Hg and unrelenting rest pain despite analgetic medication; proof that further reconstructive surgery or angioplasty was impossible by arteriography or patient condition; and the presence of nonhealing foot ulcers or dry gangrene.

Seven to 9 days after the start of iv. PGE1, the patients were randomized into receiving spinal cord stimulation (SCS) plus PGE1, the treatment group with n = 45, or just PGE1, the control group with n = 41.

Follow-up examinations and tests were done at 1, 3, 6 and 12 months.

There were no significant differences between the groups in the following: presence of diabetes, chart history of hypertension or hyperlipidemia, smoking history or habits, number or size of foot lesions, or several key group mean physiological values, including age, arm systolic or diastolic pressure, ankle systolic pressure, foot $TcPO_2$, ankle/brachial ratio (ABI), foot/chest $TcPO_2$ ratio (RPI), and walking distance. The SCS group had more prior vascular leg surgeries (1.77 vs. 1.17 per patient).

Clinical results at 12 months

There was significantly better total healing of foot ulcers in the SCS group (69 % vs. 17 %, $p < .0001$), and also better healing which was either total or at least half-way (82 % vs. 37 %, $p < .001$). Significantly more SCS patients thus achieved an outcome of Fontaine stage II (claudication pain, no rest pain or lesions) [40 % vs. 10 %, $p = .0014$] or Fontaine stage III (rest pain, no lesions) [29 % vs. 7 %, $p = .013$]. More patients in the PGE1 group had lesions, Fontaine stage IV [16 % SCS vs. 63 % PGE1, $p < .0001$]. Of patients with ulcers or wounds remaining, the SCS patients had significantly more of them heal at least half-way [86 % vs. 31 %, $p = .026$]. Mean walking distance was 84 % longer with the SCS group [337 vs. 183 meters, $p < .05$]. The frequency of minor amputations was not signi-ficantly different (13 % vs. 15 %), since all necrotic toes were eventually amputated. The frequencies of above-knee or below-knee amputations (major, foot removal) were also similar (16 % vs. 20 %), perhaps in part due to the initial use of prostaglandins on all patients. Longer follow-up may have shown a major difference, from considerations of the physiological status. Both hypertensive and normotensive patients benefited significantly from SCS, as did both diabetic and nondiabetic patients. A major finding may be that SCS improves healing of ulcers in diabetics from a 14 % rate to a 50 % rate, and cuts the risk for foot amputation by 75 %, totally offsetting this major health problem for diabetics.

Physiological results at 12 months

Foot $TcPO_2$ increased significantly for the SCS group (+213 % vs. −2 %, $p < .0001$). Patients in either group whose $TcPO_2$ rose to 26.0 ± 8.6 mm Hg on average were able to heal ulcers or toe amputation wounds. PGE1 patients had temporary $TcPO_2$ elevations of about 33 % on average due to the prostaglandin therapy, but this was gone by 6 months. SCS patients had steady increases in $TcPO_2$, and maintained them at 12 months. The RPI increased significantly (187 % vs. 0 %, $p < .001$), indicating that the $TcPO_2$ increase was in the foot skin only, not the entire circulation. The final mean ABI at 12 months of the treated limb of the SCS patients was not significantly greater, but its change from baseline was significantly larger [$+10$ % vs. -45 %, $p < .02$]. This change difference was less due to a modest increase in ABI of the SCS group, but rather a significant decline in the ABI of the OMT group ($p < .05$), the anticipated natural history of endstage PVD. Regression lines demonstrate that there is a significant improvement in "microcirculation" with SCS: on average, even when ABI was unchanged, $TcPO_2$ rose by 10.3 mm Hg = 103 % ($p < .000001$). SCS patients with initial $TcPO_2 < 10$ mm Hg did not do as well as other SCS patients in terms of complete ulcer healing (50 % vs. 84 %, $p = .023$), but they did significantly better than OMT patients with initial $TcPO_2 < 10$ mm Hg (only 5 % healing, $p = .0033$). Hence, low initial oxygen is a relative risk factor for responsiveness to SCS, but it is a compelling risk factor if SCS is not given.

Conclusion

Spinal cord stimulation appears to provide a major benefit for lesion improvement in stage IV patients with non reconstructable CLI. With pain relief and ulcer healing quality of life improved. Effects on limb salvage do not appear.

General conclusions

- SCS is effective for the relief of ischemic pain
- SCS promotes ulcer healing
- The Cologne randomized study showed no effect on limb salvage at 12 months
- Studies are mandatory to analyze the cost effectiveness
- Major complications are rare
- SCS induces an inhibition of sympathetic vasoconstrictive activity

Literature

requests: L. Claeys, MD

Author's address:
Luc Claeys MD
Dept. of Vascular Surgery
General Hospital Cologne-Porz
Urbacher Weg 19
51149 Cologne, Germany

Spinal cord stimulation (SCS) in the treatment of non-reconstructable arterial occlusive disease of upper extremities

C. Bartels, M. Bechtel, L. Claeys, K. Ktenidis, S. Horsch

Department of General and Vascular Surgery, Krankenhaus Porz am Rhein, Academic Teaching Hospital of the University of Cologne, Germany

Introduction

Ischemic vascular disease of the upper extremity is less common than peripheral arterial vascular disease of the lower limbs. Arterial occlusive vascular disease of the upper extremities as a result of severe generalized atherosclerotic disease represents a difficult therapeutic problem. In the presence of extensive distal atherosclerotic disease, arterial reconstruction is frequently impossible (15). Aggressive medical treatment has been the mainstay of treatment in these situations. Medical treatment, however, sometimes fails and tissue loss, dysfunctional limbs or major amputation may occur (16). The importance of the hand in daily living activities mandates aggressive therapeutic attempts.

Spinal cord stimulation (SCS) has been shown to be an effective therapeutic method for limb salvage, pain reduction, improvement of blood flow and healing of ulcers in severe peripheral arterial disease of the lower limbs (2, 4, 5, 7, 8, 12, 13). The efficacy of SCS for treatment of occlusive arterial disease of the upper extremity has never been evaluated. Therefore, the effect of SCS on limb salvage, pain reduction, transcutaneous oxygen tension index ($TcpO_2$ index = chest $TcpO_2$/ hand $TcpO_2$) and microcirculation in patients with severe unreconstructable peripheral occlusive arterial disease of the upper limbs was studied.

Materials and methods

Patients. All patients required strong analgetics prior to implantation of the device. In all patients the right upper extremity was the more afflicted site. Mean age of the patient cohort was 55 ± 14 years at time of implantation. In four patients ischemia was limb threatening, in three patients distal acral necrosis was present prior to implantation of the device. Patient data are summarized in Table 1.

Follow-up parameters

Parameters were assessed prior to implantation of the SCS device. After implantation, the patient was examined after the 1st week, the 1st month, the 3rd month, the 9th month, the 1st year and then at least every 12 months. All parameters were assessed after a rest period of at least 30 min in a supine position in a temperature-controlled room.

Table 1. Patients characteristics

Pat.	Age Sex	Pathologic condition	Angiographic findings	Procedures	Follow-up
1 H.K.	60 ♂	accelerated atherosclerosis of lower and upper limbs, CAD, COLD, above-knee amputation, limb-threatening ischemia, necrosis DII	occlusion of radial and ulnar artery	failed recurrent thrombectomies with intraarterial lysis and failed i.v. prostavasin, successful SCS	limb-salvage, healed necrosis, pain resolution, died of pulmonary cancer
2 S.F.	33 ♂	stab wound with occlusion of the ulnar artery, severe rest pain	thrombembolic occlusion of all major arteries by chronically occluded ulnar artery and rare collateralization	thrombectomy of brachial and radial artery with intraarterial lysis, persistent pain, successful SCS	pain resolution, minor pain at exercise
3 N.R.	47 ♀	thoracic radiation by M. Hodgin, rest pain of the right arm and hand, COLD	occlusion of the axillary artery, of the brachial and radial artery	failed thrombectomy, failed i.v. prostavasin, successful SCS	pain resolution
4 K.E.	51 ♂	stenosis of the subclavian artery, inoperable due to high operative risk, COLD, CAD, necrosis DII and DV	high grade stenosis of the subcalvian artery, occlusion of the distal digital arteries DI, DII, DV	successful SCS	healed necrosis, pain resolution
5 L.M.	60 ♂	thrombembolic occlusion of the palmar arch, rest pain, CAD, COLD	patent great arteries of the right upper extremity, occluded palmar arch	successful SCS	pain resolution
6 B.I.	54 ♂	Buerger's syndrome, severe rest pain, limb threatening ischemia, CAD, COLD	occluded ulnar artery, multiple high grade stenosis of the radial artery, partial occluded palmar arch, occlusion of all distal digital arteries	successful SCS	limb-salvage, pain resolution
7 B.A.	62 ♂	accelerated athero-sclerosis of lower and upper limbs, CAD, COLD, above-knee amputation, necrosis DIII	distal occluded radial artery, partial occluded palmar arch, occlusion of distal digital arteries DII, DIII, partial digital occlusion of DI, DIV, DV	successful SCS	pain resolution, after demarcation amputation of distal phalanx DIII, died of myocardial infarction
8 M.M.	72 ♀	accelerated athero-sclerosis of lower and upper limbs, CAD, COLD, thoracic-outlet-syndrome, limb-threatening ischemia	occlusion of all major arteries, thoracic-outlet-syndrome	sublcavian radial-ulnar bypass, chronic occluded bypass with chronic occluded major arteries, failed i.v. prostavasin, successful SCS	limb salvage, pain resolution, probe correction, infected system with explantation after 4 months
9 B.A.	38 ♂	thrombembolic occlusion of all major arteries, thoracic-outlet-syndrome, limb-threatening ischemia	chronic occluded major arteries after origin of the vertebral artery	resection of the cervical rib, failed thrombectomies, failed intraarterial lysis, successful SCS	limb-salvage, pain resolution, insertion of new probe after break of the probe
10 B.M.	75 ♀	thoracic radiation by mamma carcinoma, necrosis DI, DIII-DV, CAD, COLD	patient major arteries, occluded digital arteries	successful SCS	healed necrosis, pain resolution

age = year, CAD = coronary artery disease, COLD = chronic obstructive lung disease, D = digit, SCS = spinal cord stimulation

1. *Transcutaneous oxygen tension (TcpO₂)* was measured by the use of Clark's electrode (12). $TcpO_2$ measurements were performed at the dorsal site of both hands and at the chest wall to calculate $TcpO_2$ index (chest $TcpO_2$/hand $TcpO_2$).

2. *Pain intensity* was estimated from the patient's opinion of the degree of pain on a visual analogue scale (1 – 10; 1 = no pain) before implantation and during follow-up.

3. *Doppler wrist pressure index* was obtained (systemic systolic pressure/wrist pressure) by the use of a continuous wave Doppler device (CW-Doppler) and expressed in millimeters of mercury. Systemic systolic pressure was estimated from systolic pressure obtained by CW-Doppler measurement of an unaffected extremity. The absence of arterial affliction of these unaffected extremities was validated by findings of CW-Doppler wave amplitude, B-scan and angiography.

4. *Microcirculation* was studied for nutritional capillary morphologic characteristics and capillary blood flow by means of intravital rest capillary microscopy at the distal phalanx of both hands. The technique of capillary microscopy has been described in detail elsewhere (6). Since microcirculatory examinations were not available for all patients prior to implantation, only five patients underwent systematic microcirculatory evaluation. Dynamic capillaroscopy without dyes included the following parameters: 1) mean resting red blood cell velocity (rBCV, flying spot; normal range: 0.55 – 0.7 mm/sec), 2) capillary density (CD; normal range: 60 – 70/mm² (14). Qualitative assessment of capillary morphology was performed according to Fagrell (3).

Surgical procedure

Implantation of the electrode was performed with the patient in a prone position under local anesthesia. Under fluoroscopic control a quad-electrode (Medtronic Inc., Minneapolis, Minn.) was introduced into the epidural space at the level of C4 – C7. The surgical technique has been described in detail before (8, 10).

Statistical analysis

All data are expressed as mean values ± standard deviation (SD). Paired-sample Student's *t*-test with the Bonferroni correction was used to test statistical significance of $TcpO_2$, Doppler wrist pressure index and microcirculatory parameters. Wilcoxon test for analysis of pain intensity was performed. A p-value of less than 0.05 was considered significant.

Results

The mean follow-up was 12.8 ± 15.7 months.

Pain reduction: Spinal cord stimulation induced excellent pain reduction immediately after implantation, pain reduction remained significant during follow-up period. Exercise induced ischemic pain could be reduced effectively in all but one patient, enabling two

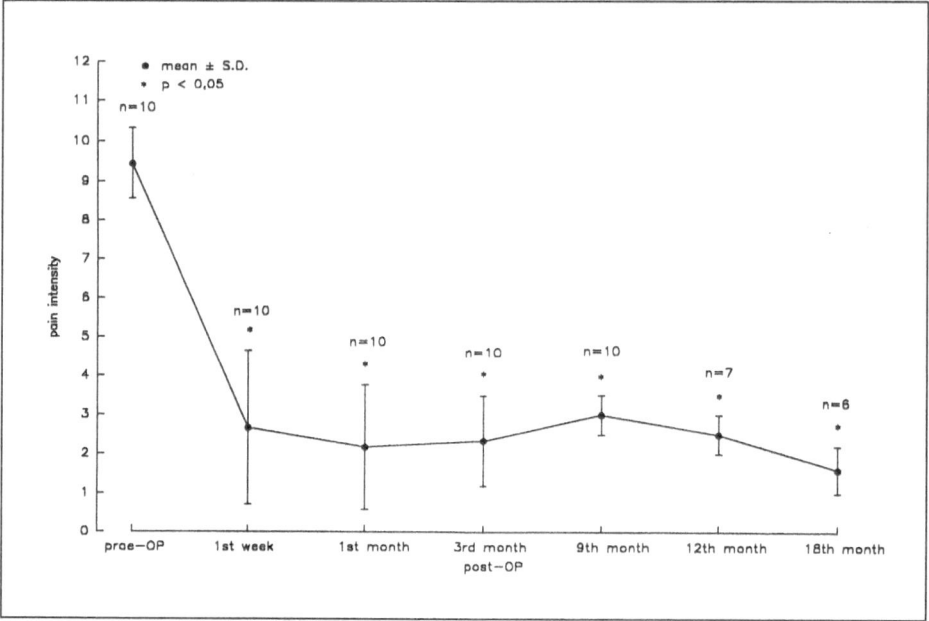

Fig. 1. Pain intensity

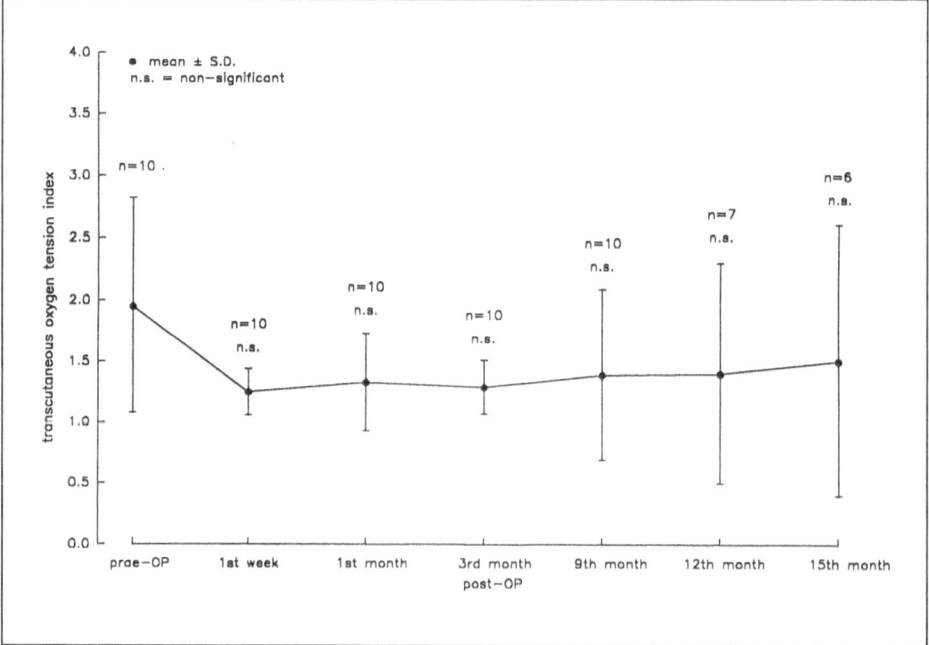

Fig. 2. Transcutaneous oxygen tension index (TcpO$_2$-index)

patients to continue their manual work. Figure 1 depicts pain reduction of the study population.

Transcutaneous oxygen tension index: $TcpO_2$ index improved insignificantly after SCS (See Fig. 2).

Doppler wrist pressure index remained unchanged throughout the follow-up period (0.2 – 1.0).

Limb-salvage: In all patients with limb-threatening ischemia the afflicted extremity could be preserved. No further distal necrosis occurred after treatment with SCS.

Microcirculation: Resting red blood cell velocity showed only a minor increase after SCS (n = 5, 0.19 ± 0.12 prior to implantation to 0.25 ± 0.23 mm/sec. after 18 months). Capillary density was not affected by treatment with SCS (n = 5, 33.75 ± 12 prior to implantation to 28.3 ± 17.6 per mm^2 at 18 months follow-up). In all patients capillary morphology was classified as Stage C according to Fagrell prior to stimulation (3). In one patient capillary morphology improved to such an extent than capillary morphology could be classified as Stage B after SCS. In the other cases amelioration was only minor and capillary morphology remained in Stage C throughout the follow-up.

Discussion

Unreconstructable severe arterial occlusive disease of the upper limbs represents a difficult therapeutic problem. Our results demonstrate that even in cases with severe limb-threatening ischemia of the upper extremity treatment with spinal cord stimulation provides limb salvage and excellent pain reduction, however, the decrease in pain intensity was not paralleled by an amelioration in microcirculatory parameters.

Vasospastic disorders of the upper extremities were successfully treated by SCS. Robiana and co-workers studied the effect of SCS on pain relief, skin temperature and peripheral blood flow in patients with primary Raynaud's disease and reflex sympathetic dystrophy (11). They experienced a good to excellent pain relief in 90 % of the patients and a concomitant increase of skin temperature and peripheral blood supply. Excellent pain relief after SCS was observed in seven patients with vasospastic disorders of the upper extremity by Augustinsson and co-workers (1). More recently, excellent pain reduction and improvement of skin blood flow has been reported by our group in a larger patient collective (n = 177) with unreconstructable arterial occlusive disease of the lower limbs treated by SCS (5). Fiume et al. and Sciacca et al. observed a significant increase of $TcpO_2$ in patients with PAD of the legs treated by SCS (4, 12). These and other studies demonstrated that the treatment of ischemic vascular disease by SCS decreases pain intensity and improves blood supply, assessed by different methods (4, 8, 12, 13).

In contrast to these results no improvement of microcirculatory parameters could be observed in the studied patients with severe arterial occlusive disease of the upper limbs. How can this unexpected result be explained?

1) Most clinical studies use the measurement of $TcpO_2$ for determination of skin blood flow (4, 12). Nevertheless, as the skin $TcpO_2$ reflects systemic changes, e.g., pulmonary gas exchange, cardiac output even a $TcpO_2$ index (chest $TcpO_2$/hand $TcpO_2$) may be altered by pathologic conditions of the cardiovascular and/or pulmonary function. 70 % of the studied patients suffered from cardiovascular and pulmonary disease.

2) Improvement of dynamic microcirculatory parameters after treatment with SCS has been observed by Jacobs et al. in patients with PAD of the lower limbs (8). Since red blood cell velocity (rBCV) and capillary density (CD) may reflect changes in the nutritional blood flow, these parameters may be more reliable for assessment of blood supply in ischemic limbs than changes in $TcpO_2$ index (8). Only a minor improvement of rBCV could be observed in the studied five patients; CD remained constant after treatment with SCS. However, the lack of a statistically significant increase in rBCV and CD seems to be related to the small number of studied patients and the inhomogeneous patient group. As expected, only minor improvements were observed concerning the classification of Fagrell. Further studies with a larger and more homogeneous patient collective are warranted to study the effect of SCS on dynamic and qualitative capillary microscopic parameters.

In most cases reconstructive surgery of arterial occlusive disease of the upper extremity is feasible, however surgery may be impossible in some cases (15). More recently arteriovenous reversal in six upper extremities with arterial occlusive disease due to vasospastic and atherosclerotic disease has been performed with good results regarding limb salvage and pain relief (9). However, only two patients of this collective suffered from atherosclerotic disease, the remaining patients had an underlying vasospastic disease. In all patients with vasospastic disease a patent radial artery was present prior to arteriovenous reversal, this condition may explain the good surgical results. In our patient group, angiography demonstrated in 50 % of the patients chronic occlusion of major arteries or major atherosclerotic changes which suggests that arteriovenous reversal in these cases might not be comparably successful. In four of these patients limb-threatening ischemia was present prior to SCS, in all cases the extremity could be preserved and rest pain disappeared.

In patients with severe PAD of the upper limbs not amenable to revascularisation procedures and failed conservative treatment, SCS should be considered as an alternative therapeutic method for limb-salvage and pain reduction.

References

1. Augustinsson LE, Holm J, Carlsson AC, Jivegard L (1985) Epidural electrical stimulation in severe limb ischemia. Evidence of pain relief, increased blood flow and a possible limb-saving effect. Ann Surg 202: 104–111
2. Claeys L, Ktenidis K, Horsch S (1994) Transcutaneous oxygen tension in patients with critical limb ischemia treated by spinal cord stimulation. In: Horsch S, Claeys L (eds). Spinal cord stimulation. Darmstadt, Berlin, Heidelberg, New York, London, Paris: Steinkopff: 145–152
3. Fagrell B (1990) Techniques and normal findings. In: Bollinger A, Fagrell B (eds). Clinical capillaroscopy. Toronto, New York: Hogrefe and Huber: 1–9
4. Fiume D, Palombi M, Sciacca V, Tamorri M (1989) Spinal cord stimulation in peripheral ischemic pain. Pace 12: 698–704
5. Horsch S, Claeys L (1994) Epidural spinal cord stimulation in the treatment of severe peripheral arterial occlusive disease. Ann Vasc Surg 8: 468–474
6. Jacobs MJHM, Breslau PJ, Slaaf DW, Reneman RS, Lemmens HAJ (1987) Nomenclature of Raynaud's phenomenon. A capillary microscopic and hemorheologic study. Surgery 101: 136–145
7. Jacobs MJHM, Jörning PJG, Joshi SR, Kitslaar PJEHM, Slaaf DW, Reneman RS (1988) Epidural spinal cord electrical stimulation improves microvascular blood flow in severe limb ischemia. Ann Surg 207: 179–183
8. Jacobs MJHM, Jörning PJG, Beckers RJG et al. (1990) Foot salvage and improvement of microvascular blood flow as a result of epidural spinal cord electrical stimulation. J Vasc Surg 12: 354–360

9. King TA, Marks J, Berrettoni BA, Seitz WH (1993) Arteriovenous reversal for limb salvage in unreconstructable upper extremity arterial occlusive disease. J Vasc Surg 17: 924–933
10. Ktenidis K, Claeys L, Horsch S (1994) Epidural spinal cord stimulation (ESCS): implantation technique. In: Horsch S, Claeys L (eds) Spinal cord stimulation. Darmstadt, Berlin, Heidelberg, New York, London, Paris. Steinkopff: 75–82
11. Robaina FJ, Dominguez M, Diaz M, Rodriguez JL, de Vera JA (1989) Spinal cord stimulation for relief of chronic pain in vasospastic disorders of the upper limbs. Neurosurgery 24: 63–67
12. Sciacca V, Mingoli A, Di Marzo L, Maggiore C, Fiume D, Cavallaro A (1989) Predictive value of transcutaneous oxygen tension measurement in the indication for spinal cord stimulation in patients with peripheral vascular disease: preliminary results. Vasc Surg 23: 128–132
13. Tallis RC, Illis LS, Sedgwick EM, Hardwidge C, Garfield JS (1983) Spinal cord stimulation in peripheral vascular disease. J Neurol Neurosurg Psychiatry 46: 478–484
14. Tyml K, Ellis CG (1982) Evaluation of the flying spot technique as a television method for measuring red cell velocities in microvessels. Int J Micocirc Clin Exp 1: 145–155
15. Whitehouse WM (1984) Direct revascularisation for forearm and hand ischemia. In: Bergan JJ, Yao JST (eds). Evaluation and treatment of upper and lower extremity circulatory disorders. New York: Grune and Stratton
16. Yao JST, McDaniel MD, King TA (1984) Arterial surgery of the upper extremity. In: Bergan JJ (ed) Clinical surgery international: arterial surgery. London: Churchill Livingstone, pp 201–224

Author's address:
Claus Bartels, MD
Department of Vascular Surgery
Acad. Teach.-Hospital
Univ. of Cologne
Urbacher Weg 19
51149 Köln, Germany

Spinal cord stimulation (SCS): a convenient enrichment or an expensive adventure in vascular surgery?

H. M. Becker*, K. Ktenidis**

 * Department of Vascular Surgery, Academic Teaching Hospital München-Neuperlach, University of
   Munich, Germany
** Department of General and Vascular Surgery, Krankenhaus Porz am Rhein, Academic Teaching
   Hospital of the University of Cologne, Germany

In present times it is vital to always consider cost compared to therapeutic gain when new treatment methods are introduced to medicine. The new method has to be critically judged in order to prove adequate superiority to what is available. However, new concepts are often introduced as additional therapy rather than replacing older renowned methods, and for this reason a true comparison is rather difficult due to ethical reasons. Only few studies have succeeded to assess cost and use of various therapies individually.

Indication

Stimulation of the spinal cord using electric currents is an example of a new therapeutic availability to avoid amputations in critical limb ischemia due to peripheral vascular disease (La Fontaine classification stage III or IV). Implantation of the mentioned device is considered justified when vascular reconstruction has failed or is impossible, and an amputation in the near future is inevitable.

Cost-use analysis of limb salvaging and amputatory procedures

The first detailed prospective cost-analysis in PVD patients with severe limb ischemia was performed by Bruijnen and Loeprecht in 1989, who assessed the total cost of in-hospital treatment for peripheral vascular disease. Indication for admission to hospital was an ulcerated leg ischemia (La Fontaine Stage IV). The post-operative mortality over the first 6 months was 17 %. Patients, whose limb could be salvaged, accumulated an average minimum cost of DM 13562. An amputation, occasionally preceeded by futile vascular reconstruction averaged an expenditure of DM 22946 per patient, or DM 25364 considering all patients in total (Table 1).

The authors determined the cost for patients who survived the early post-operative stage after limb salvage to be DM 14069, for those who were amputated after futile vascular reconstruction at DM 27583, and the cost of primary amputation at an average of DM 28186 per patient.

Table 1. Comparison of average cost in DM

	Total	Surviving patients
Limb salvage	13 562	14 069
Limb loss	25 364	27 583
Primary amputation	22 946	28 186

Raviola et al. (8) analyzed the hospitalization costs for femoro-popliteal bypass operations (n = 94) and primary amputations (n = 53) in 1988. The average cost of the uncomplicated bypass was $ 20 300 compared to $ 14 000 for uncomplicated below-knee amputations. However, the total cost of the amputation including rehabilitation and prosthesis was $ 20 400. If a complication arose after BKA, the hospital stay usually lengthened by an average of 12.5 days increasing costs to a total of $ 40 600. Complications requiring reintervention after the initial bypass only lengthened hospital stays by 4.5 days on average and the cost rose to $ 28 700 per patient.

Mackey et al. (7) in 1986 reported the long-term cost analysis of primary amputations versus initial vascular reconstruction in a follow-up period of 805 ± 57 days the average expenditure for vascular reconstruction was $ 40 769 ± 3726. 28 high-risk patients were treated by primary amputation at an average cost of $ 40 563 ± 4729 in a follow-up period of 663 ± 97 days (7).

Every effort to avoid amputation at high medical and economic cost as well as a satisfactory rehabilitation is considered the worthwhile aim in the mentioned studies. Neurostimulation can achieve a markedly more distal amputation level or even negate the necessity of an amputation.

Horsch et al. (4) claim a 5-year-limb preservation rate of 85 % in stage III disease (n = 169) and 43 % in stage IV (n = 68) disease. Additionally, a significant improvement in the $TcpO_2$ value from 24.8 mmHg to 48.1 mmHg determined on the dorsal foot was recorded in stage III, and from 15.44 mmHg to 37.6 mmHg in stage IV patients (4). More than 80 % of patients with stage III disease (n = 114) also described a significant pain reduction in the affected limb. "Significant pain reduction" was understood to be a reduction of more than 75 % using the visual analogue scale pre- and post operatively.

Table 2 presents the financial aspect to the spinal cord stimulator. The cost of the complete set is DM 13 100.

Implantation requires a hospital stay of merely 3 days. The procedure is performed under local anaesthetic and can be completed on the day of admission if preoperative preparations are performed on an out-patient basis. The patient is restricted to 24 h bedrest after implantation and after this the spinal cord stimulator is programmed. Should the stimulation be satisfactory (pleasant paraesthesias in the affected limb and a feeling of warmth), the patient can be dismissed into out-patient care on the second postoperative day.

Table 2. Average cost of spinal cord stimulation (DM)

Cost of hospitalization (3 days)	1 200
Cost of the complete system	13 100
Total sum	14 300

Conclusion

An average of 30000 major amputations is performed in Germany every year, causing an escalation of hospital costs into the millions. This becomes apparent in the brief presentation of the aforementioned studies. The unanimous opinion of all studies is that preservation of a limb is the most cost-effective treatment for PVD patients from a medical as well as economic point of view.

Spinal cord stimulation is able to increase the limb preservation rate as well as decrease the consumption of analgetics for intractable pain. The first question, whether spinal cord stimulation enriches vascular surgery with new treatment options, can be undisputedly agreed upon.

The second question, whether this is an expensive adventure in vascular surgery, requires a differentiated denial.

If the indication for implantation is carefully set and applied in a selective approach, the presently high costs of the system can be justified by the middle and long-term success rates. (Reduction of amputation rate and analgetic consumption.) The differentiated denial now turns into a definite no.

References

1. Augustinsson LE, Carlsson CA, Holm J, Jivegård L (1985) Pidural electrical stimulation in severe limb ischemia. In: Surg 202: 104–110
2. Bruijnen H, Loeprecht H (1989) Kosten. Nutzen-Analyse der Beinerhaltung. Langenbecks Arch Chir Suppl II: 617–619
3. Claeys L, Ktenidis K, Horsch S (1994) Trancutaneous Oxygen tension in patients with critical limb ischemia treated by spinal cord stimulation. In: Horsch S, Claeys L. Spinal Cord Stimulation. Steinkopff Verlag, Darmstadt, pp 145
4. Horsch S, Claeys L, Ktenidis K (1993) Epidurale Rückenmarksstimulation beim austherapierten arteriellen Verschlußleiden. Langenbecks Arch Chir, Suppl 580–585
5. Jacobs MJHM (1994) Vascular disease and spinal cord stimulation. In: Horsch S, Claeys L. Spinal Cord Stimulation. Steinkopff Verlag, Darmstadt, pp 153
6. Kasprzak P, Raithel D (1994) Can spinal cord stimulation reduce the amputation rate in patient with critical limb ischemia? In: Horsch S, Claeys L. Spinal Cord Stimulation. Steinkopff Verlag, Darmstadt, pp 165
7. Mackey WC, McCullough JL, Conton TP, Shepard AD, Deterling RA, Callow Ad, O'Donnel TF (1986) The costs of surgery for limb-treatening ischemia. Surgery 99: 26–35
8. Raviola CA, Nichter LS, Baker JD, Busuttil RW, Machleder HI, Moore WS (1988) Cost of treating advanced leg ischemia. Arch Surg 123: 495–9

Author's address:
Prof. Hans-Martin Becker, MD, PhD
Chief of Vascular Surgery
Hospital München-Neuperlach
Oskar-Maria-Graf-Ring 51
81737 München, Germany

Carotid surgery – past, present and future

P. Panoussis

Department of Vascular Surgery, "KAT" General Hospital, Athens, Greece

Medicine, at the end of the twentieth century, encompasses the period of its great achievements.

Carotid artery surgery is a branch of vascular surgery which has developed mostly in the past few years. There is a great number of new strokes each year, and death is the eventual outcome in about 1/3 of these cases. As a result, cerebrovascular accidents are the third leading cause of death worldwide, following coronary artery disease and cancer. In addition, there is a very great number of stroke patients alive but unfortunately disabled.

First of all, we must note that in medical knowledge almost everything is connected with ancient Greece. The word "carotid" has derived from the ancient Greek word "carossis". Its first meaning was to stupefy or plunge into a deep sleep. The 31st metope of the south side of the Parthenon in Athens is now situated in the British Museum, in London, among the other Greek marbles carried there by Elgin; it demonstrates that ancient Greeks were aware of the left carotid compression on the neck of a Lapith warrior. The Centaurs were wild men of Thessaly, who came to be depicted as half men and half horses. In the Centaur battles, they knew the great significance of the carotid artery. They knew that if they managed to compress the artery, they would send their enemy to deep sleep, and defeat him. This retrospection to ancient Greek history helps us to understand the history of the word "carotid".

Ambroise Paré in the sixteenth century called these vessels "the right and left carotides or sleepy arteries". Also, it is remarkable that Hippocrates and Galenos were aware that hemiplegia resulted from a lesion in the opposite side of the brain.

In the eighteenth century, it was observed that the function of the brain might be normal, even if one carotid was totally obliterated.

Thomas Willis declared that the circle of Willis was complete in most people and capable of sustaining adequate blood flow to the brain through only one of the four normal inflow vessels. The suggestion that the etiology of stroke was intracranial persisted for almost 250 years. In the 1930s, in careful cadaveric dissections, Miller-Abbott identified a complete circle of Willis in only 25 % of cadavers. The remainder had many variations, but adequate blood flow would not likely be possible with one -vessel inflow alone. However, it took the advent of angiography to link extracranial vascular disease with stroke or transient neurological events.

With new anatomic information available, surgical judgement dictated that the eradication of a plaque at the carotid bifurcation should reduce the risk of stroke. The basis of this surgical judgement was the growing success with other vascular surgical procedures and an increasing awareness of a role for atherosclerotic plaque, as the potential cause of local and distant disease.

In 1954, the first carotid endarterectomy was performed, although it was done under circumstances that would not be appropriate today, in that the patient was suffering from a stroke in evolution. However, this bold venture stimulated interest in the procedure. Experience was gained with respect to operative survival and patient benefit. The indications for operation were based on the carefully considered advantages and disadvantages for each patient, without formal statistical interference.

There was a relatively slow general acceptance of this procedure. However, the inquisitive surgical mind combined with increased surgical abilities led to an accelerated increase in the number of endarterectomies performed. This was linked to the training of neurosurgeons and vascular surgeons capable of performing the procedure and the burgeoning of noninvasive technology to identify patients with carotid artery disease.

The enthusiasm for carotid endarterectomies continued unabated until the mid-1980s, when the number of endarterectomies had risen considerably annually, making it the second most common surgical procedure performed in all vascular units.

In the mid-1980s, a report was released stating that the extracranial intracranial bypass procedure did not reduce the risk of stroke, when added to maximum medical therapy. This was a large multicenter trial, and the negative results had a devastating impact upon a number of neurological centers that had built a future around cerebral revascularization. For vascular surgeons, the nature of that specific intervention did not have the same compelling rationale as eradication of an offending plaque within the extracranial circulation.

In this climate of uncertainty the North American Symptomatic Carotid Endarterectomy Trial (known as NASCET) was proposed as a randomized prospective trial. The question asked was: Does the addition of carotid endarterectomy to maximum medical therapy significantly reduce the risk of stroke? This was an open challenge to surgeons: Had their judgement been correct in the past, and were they capable of performing this procedure with a low complication rate?

It is to the credit of vascular surgeons that many embraced this study with enthusiasm and made major contributions to its eventual success. The results of the NASCET could not have been more positive for surgery. The trial was terminated prematurely because the medically managed group had a much higher than predicted rate of strokes, certainly much higher than it had previously been reported in medical trials.

These results were valid in a specific subset of patients whose stenosis was greater than 70 %, who had symptoms less than 120 days before their operation and who were appropriate surgical candidates. For these patients, carotid endarterectomy definitely reduced the risk of stroke. Within this group, surgical intervention had become relatively straightforward and virtually without contention.

Surgical judgement that led the carotid endarterectomy as a procedure for stroke prevention must now be applied in the light of the understanding we have gained from the NASCET. That trial has not answered all the questions concerning carotid endarterectomy. Although we know that carotid endarterectomy is applicable to a certain subgroup of patients with stroke symptoms and extracranial vascular disease, it is not absolutely contraindicated for all other patients, nor can this information be applied globally to any patients with extracranial vascular occlusive disease. The basis for effective surgical decision making also relates to the details of surgical technique and the application of this knowledge to specific conditions.

In cerebrovascular insufficiency morbidity at times may be more important than mortality, thus the quality of survival is emphasized as the future of this disease, and underlines the main role of carotid endarterectomy as one of stroke prevention.

We must finally hope and wish that the studies today will show that high-risk groups benefit from carotid surgery. Unfortunately, these trials will not solve all problems, because they take into consideration only the degree of stenosis, although it is very possible that the morphology of the stenosis, the atheromatic plaque, is determinant in the decision of therapy. At present, although there is great progress in echo-Doppler and IRM, it is not yet possible to ignore an asymptomatic high-risk group, that would justify surgical intervention, based on the morphological characteristics of the atheromatic plaque.

Finally, it seems that there are still many problems that need solution in carotid end-arterectomy, and we hope to find some answers in this Greek-German Symposium. One of these problems is the kind of anesthesia. It has never been proved that local anesthesia has been of benefit in carotid surgery. In fact, it concerns only some special cases. In addition, the perioperative monitoring, the indications of a shunt, the operative angiography, the sort of closure of the arteriotomy constitute the personal choice and habit of the surgical team. The only important thing is of course the final result of a correct geometry of carotid occlusion.

In conclusion, I would like to say that carotid surgery has improved significantly. Neurologists from all over Europe including Greece are in favor of surgery under the existing conditions, with the ulterior purpose to keep the light of the mind of the patient on, his eyes open, and the smile on his face, and to prevent the thunder of the stroke.

References

1. Bergquist D (1994) Risk benefit aspects of surgery for symptomatic carotid stenosis. International symposium "Risk Benefit Aspects of Vascular Surgery". Stockholm, Sweden, May 1994
2. Boardman J, Finn D (1985) The Parthenon and its sculptures. Thames and Hudson Ltd, 1985, London
3. Ruckley CV, Wildsmith JAW (1992) Carotid endarterectomies: future perspectives. Eur J Vasc Surg 6: 229-231
4. Thompson JE (1986) History of carotid artery surgery. Surg Clin of North America. Vol 66, No 2

Author's address:
Prof. Panos Panoussis
"KAT" General Hospital of Athens
2, Nikis St.
14561 Kifisia-Athens, Greece

Diagnostic methods in carotid surgery

D. Velecheris

Department of Radiology, "IKA" Hospital, Athens, Greece

One of the main characteristics of the clinical picture of stenosis or occlusion of the carotid artery is the variety of pathological findings.

The extent of the lesion in the cerebral tissue depends on the state of the anastomotic circulation of the cerebral arteries. The development of different neurogical deficits (amaurosis fugax, transient ischemic attack, progressive stroke, completed stroke) also depends on this.

In other cases this is possible when there is a gradual developing stenosis which finally leads to occlusion without any symptoms (asymptomatic cases of carotid disease).

Stroke is defined as a clinical syndrome of neurological findings whose vascular origins are limited to occlusion or rupture of a cerebral artery.

Occlusion generally stems from primary intracranial thrombosis or by secondary embolism from an extracranial site producing regional ischemia and infarction (cardiac abnormalities, carotid stenosis-occlusion, plaque rupture, intraplaque hemorrhage crater formalism thrombosis).

Arterial rupture produces intraparenchymal or subarachnoid hemorrhage resulting in ischemia by interrupting the regional blood supply from spasm or compression of local tissue.

Rare cases of malformation of the carotid arteries have been noted (Megadolicho carotid arteries, aneurysm trauma, Takayasus disease, carotid cavernous fistulae, tumors, syphon stenosis). This may cause a number of cerebral disturbances (sudden deafness, persistent pharyngeal discomfort, sudden hemiplegia, rupture, death, etc.).

The following is an overview of various diagnostic techniques that provide information on the existing carotid disease as well as indication for a successful operation (e.g., the non-existence stenotic lesions on the basilar cerebral arteries including the circle of Willis).

There is no doubt that routine examination of the elderly would disclose significant carotid disease in many cases but would lead to a dilemma of therapy. Autopsy studies have shown that carotid disease is very common, even in asymptomatic patients.

Clinical examination

Through clinical examination can be detected:
a) Carotid Bruit (must be differentiated from venous hum valvular stenosis, vascular disease in the great vessels, anemia, thyrotoxicosis arteriovenous malformation). A Carotid Bruit is accurately localized over the carotid bifurcation resulting from audible turbulence.
b) Palpable mass on the neck.

c) Cholesterol emboli (detected on routine ophthalmic examination, appears as bright plaques caused by cholesterol fragments associated with embolization from an atheromatous lesion and may be the first indication of significant atherosclerosis.

Diagnostic methods

Diagnostic methods used for carotid examination:
a) Carotid Bruit
b) A typical TIA
c) Monitoring progression of known disease
d) Follow-up postendarterectory
   prior to major vascular surgery
e) Cholesterol emboli
f) Routine examination of the elderly

The degree of stenosis, plaque morphology, intraplaque hemorrhage and collateral circulation all influence the clinical importance of a carotid lesion.

The diagnostic methods are invasive and noninvasive.

Noninvasive tests are widely used as the primary method of assessing patients with symptoms of cerebral ischemia. In some cases, noninvasive tests are the only method of assessment of the carotid artery before carotid endarterectomy. The ideal noninvasive test should have the ability to identify the normal carotid bifurcation, all ranges of stenotic disease, including occlusion, surface and structural characteristics of the plaque. It should do so with no risk to the patient and it should be cost effective.

Carotid lesions may be studied by examining the plaque itself or the hemodynamic changes caused by the lesion. Noninvasive tests of the cerebral circulation can be classified as direct or indirect. Direct tests detect disease at its anatomic location on the basis of local flow changes and plaque characteristics. Indirect tests determine the presence of disease by detecting hemodynamic changes at some distance from the lesion (usually the periorbital circulation).

The indirect noninvasive tests for carotid artery disease are no longer acceptable because of the high risk of a poor diagnosis. Periorbital Doppler examination can be helpful as a confirmatory test for severe disease or complete occlusion. As the pressure in the

Table 1. Invasive – noninvasive testing methods

Invasive	Noninvasive tests for carotid artery disease	
	Direct tests	Indirect tests
Angiography C.T. angiography	1. Continuous wave Doppler ultrasonography 2. Doppler spectral analysis 3. Transcranial Doppler ultrasonography 4. Real-time B-mode imaging ultrasonography 5. Duplex ultrasonography (with or without color Doppler) 6. Magnetic resonance angiography (MRA)	1. Periorbital Doppler ultrasonography 2. Oculoplethysmography

terminal branches of the ophthalmic, the supratrochlear and supraorbital arteries falls because of either complete or near occlusion, flow becomes reversed, since the pressure in the anastomosing branches from the facial and superficial temporal arteries becomes greater than the ophthalmic branches. Thus the direction of flow in the supraorbital and supratrochlear vessels reverses into the cranium. Authors reported a sensitivity of 50–90 % of this method and a specificity of 70–80 %.

C.W. Doppler ultrasound gives no axial resolution and therefore accurate anatomic localization of signals is not possible.

Continuous-wave Doppler scanning may be useful in carotid evaluation. However pulsed Doppler ultrasound is a very valuable addition. The ability to accurately locate the origin of the signal in relation to its position in the lumen enhances the diagnostic accuracy of the duplex scan. Some operators use C.W. while tracing the course of the carotid arteries, and then use pulsed Doppler ultrasound to locate the maximum peak velocity most accurately, since this peak velocity may be limited to a small pinhole in the vessel lumen.

Spectral analysis of the Doppler audio signal has considerably increased the performance accuracy of the Doppler examination. By means of the audio signal and velocity curve of C.W. Doppler it is possible to detect stenosis > 60 % by area. By spectral analysis of the Doppler audio signal it is possible to detect hemodynamic disturbances caused by stenosis of 15 % by area and to quantity higher degrees of stenosis according to the amplitude of the spectrum disturbance.

The comparison between spectral and angiographic findings showed an agreement in 68 % of the cases and 15 % false positive findings. Spectral analysis and C.W. Doppler are very simple to use and very accurate for the evaluation of carotid stenosis, but they must be performed by skilled Doppler operators.

Transcranial Doppler ultrasonography

Transcranial Doppler ultrasonography is complementary to duplex ultrasonography in the assessment of cerebral blood flow. With a low-frequency (2 MHz) pulsed Doppler beam, the skull can be penetrated and the intracranial vessels assessed, and this has led to broad application of the test in the fields of neuro and vascular surgery.

The technique utilizes a number of identified acoustic windows in the skull to examine all the vessels and major branches of the circle of Willis, including the middle cerebral

Table 2. Criteria for degrees of stenosis with spectral classification in five grades

Grade I	Stenosis < 40 % in area	Stenosis < 23 % in diameter
Grade II	Stenosis of 40–60 % in area	Stenoses of 23 to 40 % in diameter
Grade III	Extended stenoses of 60 to 75 % in area	Extended stenoses of 40 to 50 % in diameter
Grade IV	Extended stenoses of 75 to 90 % in area	Short stenoses of 60 to 90 % in area
Grade V	Stenoses > 90 % in area	Stenoses > 70 % in diameter

artery, the anterior and posterior communicating arteries, the basilar artery and the intracranial internal carotid arteries. Four different approaches to these vessels have been described: transtemporal, transorbital, suboccipital and submandibular. Vessels are identified according to the window or foramina used, the angulation of the beam, the depth of intonation, the direction of blood flow and the traceability of the vessel segments.

Areas of intracranial stenosis show localized velocity increases with turbulence. Vasospasm also shows velocity increase, but these tend to be generalized. Vessel occlusion is diagnosed by an absence of flow in an area where a particular vessel is expected to be, or a damped waveform can be caused proximal to the site of recording intracranial vascular (arteriovenous malformations, etc.) bruits or musical murmurs, associated with higher than normal velocities and flow disturbances. This diagnosis is difficult and requires an experienced examiner.

A duplex examination must be carried out before assessment of intracranial stenosis so that the status of the extracranial vessels is known. Transcranial Doppler ultrasonography can identify intracranial vessel stenosis and occlusion in patients with ischemic cerebrovascular symptoms. The accuracy of the technique has not been well documented, and arteries are generally classified as being normal, having hemodynamically significant stenosis or being occluded. Transcranial Doppler ultrasonography is particularly useful in the patient with ischemic cerebrovascular symptoms and normal findings on extracranial duplex ultrasonography, and in patients with vertebrobasilar symptoms. The technique may also be helpful in the patient being considered for carotid endarterectomy without angiography.

Transcranial Doppler ultrasonography can access the collateral flow in patients with extracranial occlusive disease. The patency of the circle of Willis can be determined. The response of distal vessels (e.g., the middle cerebral artery) to carotid artery or vertebral artery compression can be assessed. The relevance of collateral flow identified by transcranial Doppler ultrasonography to prognosis or operative planning is uncertain.

Transcranial Doppler ultrasonography has been used to monitor middle cerebral artery flow during carotid endarterectomy. Decreased flow velocity with carotid clamping suggests a need for shunting the carotid artery. A decrease of flow velocity in the middle cerebral artery of 65 % or a velocity of less than 10 cm/s is necessary to alter somatosensory-evoked potentials. Flow above these limits likely represents adequate collateral flow, but these parameters have not been tested clinically to date.

Real time B-mode imaging

The Doppler imaging techniques diagrammatically recreate the vessel lumen on a storage oscilloscope when flow velocity exceeds threshold values. Doppler imaging also provides a direct evaluation, but it is based upon the physiology of flow.

Real-time B-mode ultrasonic imaging provides structural detail of the vessel wall and atherosclerotic plaque.

Questions quickly arose as to whether important characteristics of the atheroma could be identified, specifically plaque ulceration and subintimal hemorrhage.

In determining sensitivity and specificity of the method, arteriography was the standard used to judge the noninvasive study. As any noninvasive study approaches a 90 % specificity or sensitivity, the reliability of arteriography may limit any further improvement by the noninvasive study because of the inconsistencies of arteriography. While it is well accepted that arteriograms can relatively reliably identify the normal and the highly diseased vessels, it has been clearly shown that arteriography does not reliably identify moderate disease.

Real-time B-mode ultrasonic imaging without Doppler shows only a part of the vessel wall without structural detail of the whole vessel and its flow. Duplex ultrasonography provides not only information regarding the degree of stenosis, but also gives an ultrasonic characterisation of the plaque.

Duplex ultrasonography

Duplex ultrasonography is the most useful noninvasive test for cerebrovascular disease. Old indirect tests are not as accurate.

Duplex ultrasonography was first developed for the investigation of carotid bifurcation disease by Barber and assistants in 1974, because of the perceived shortcomings of imaging and pulsed Doppler methods when used separately. The Doppler technique can provide important flow-related data but is of limited value unless the sampled site and angle of intonation is known. The ultrasonic image may provide important morphologic information but may not distinguish thrombus and is inaccurate in classifying the degree of stenosis. The combination of B-mode and Doppler ultrasonography overcomes many of the individual limitations of each technique. There have been marked improvements in the reliability, availability and accuracy of the technology, including the development of color Doppler ultrasonography, since the introduction of duplex ultrasonography. Color assignments are based on the direction and velocity of flow (i.e., varying shades of red for arterial and blue for venous flow velocities).

An over-reliance on the color Doppler signal can lead to errors. The color signal is not angle-corrected, so changes in vessel direction in relation to the scan head can cause

Table 3. Classification of internal carotid artery stenosis

Classification	Description
Normal	Internal carotid peak systolic velocity ≤ 120 cm/s No spectral broadening during the deceleration phase of systole Presence of boundary layer separation in the carotid bulb
Minimal stenosis, 1–15 % diameter reduction	Internal carotid peak systolic velocity ≤ 120 cm/s Minimal spectral broadening
Moderate stenosis, 16–49 % diameter reduction	Internal carotid peak systolic velocity $\leq$ cm/s Spectral broadening with filling of the systolic window
Severe stenosis, 50–79 % diameter reduction	Internal carotid peak systolic velocity > 120 cm/s Marked spectral broadening and posted stenotic
Critical stenosis, 80–99 % diameter reduction	Internal carotid peak systolic velocity > 120 cm/s Internal carotid end-diastolic velocity > 135 cm/s
Complete occlusion	No flow signal in an adequately visualized internal carotid artery with characteristic low or reversed flow in the common carotid artery

changes in color assignment suggesting stenosis when none is present. Even in relatively straight vessels, reliance on color Doppler ultrasonography to diagnose stenosis can lead to errors. There are, to date, no quantitative color Doppler criteria that accurately identify carotid stenosis. Steinke, Kloetzsch and Hennerici, in a comparison of duplex ultrasonography, color Doppler ultrasonography and angiography, were able to show an accuracy of 92 % to 96 % for color Doppler ultrasonography, but this was based on subjective assessment only of the color image and also utilized Doppler calculated flow velocities.

There is a wide variety of methods for the classification of carotid disease based on duplex ultrasonography assessment. Most are based on empirical comparison with arteriography. Only a few have been validated prospectively.

Various other parameters have been suggested for the classificafion of carotid artery disease, including systolic velocity ratios in the internal and common carotid arteries, end-diastolic velocity, peak diastolic velocity and diastolic velocity rations.

Some authors suggest that B-mode characteristics such as plaque hemorrhage, calcification and ulceration are important, and they carefully look for and report these findings. There are, however, conflicting results about which ultrasonography findings correlate with the pathologic findings, and the ultrasonography characteristics used to determine these features remain subjective.

The criteria base disease classification on evidence of spectral broadening for stenosis of less than 50 % diameter reduction and on velocity increases in the area of the stenosis for stenoses greater than 50 % diameter reduction. For critical stenoses of more than 80 % diameter reduction, increased end-diastolic velocity is used as a further criterion. In normal arteries, the finding of boundary-layer separation in the carotid bulb is expected.

The overall accuracy of these criteria is 82 % when compared with that of angiography. The ability to recognize normal arteries (specificity) is 84 %, and the sensitivity is 99 %. Most errors are in distinguishing normal arteries from those with minimal disease. The distinction is rarely clinically important.

Duplex ultrasonography has an important role to play in patients with asymptomatic carotid artery stenosis. Asymptomatic patients who may be candidates for carotid endarterectomy must be identified with noninvasive testing, because it is not clinically or economically feasible to access them initially by angiography. Also, in all the studies predicting risk of stroke in asymptomatic patients, it is the duplex ultrasonographic criteria alone that predict stroke risk, not the degree of stenosis determined subsequently by angiography. Angiographically measured stenosis may not be as clinically relevant as duplex ultrasonographic criteria in asymptomatic patients.

Magnetic resonance angiography

Magnetic resonance imaging is beginning to be applied to the assessment of the flow characteristics of the carotid circulation and to a determination of the degree of stenosis. The technique is widely available but because of high equipment costs its availability is limited.

MR angiography is an attractive option at first sight because it is noninvasive and avoids the hazards of contrast injection and x-ray.

In this technique, areas of flowing blood can be made to appear "bright" or "dark" by magnetic resonance imaging according to relative proton excitation. The images can be acquired by a two-dimensional or three-dimensional method for subsequent display. Final images appear similar to the familiar format of standard carotid angiography. One advantage of magnetic resonance angiography is that the brain parenchyma can be imaged at the same examination.

The accuracy of this method of assessing carotid stenosis is steadily improving. Accuracy in the detection of carotid artery stenosis greater than 50 % ranges from 69 % to 91 % in reported series. Most errors associated with magnetic resonance angiography are related to overestimation of the degree of stenosis when compared with standard angiography. In normal subjects, flow voids are seen in the carotid bifurcation. Turbulence and retrograde flow result in black holes on MRA. MR has also difficulty in distinguishing high-grade stenosis from occlusion. Two-and three-dimensional time of flight (TOF) and phase contrast MRA techniques continue to improve and may become the standard for diagnosis, but cannot be seen as such today. Without proper improvements and further clinical studies MRA has the risk of unfulfilled expectations, analogous to i.v. DSA. On the other hand, MRA has the potential to develop into a noninvasive technique that can provide anatomical and functional information about the extra- and intracranial vessels. At the present stage, it has sufficient specificity to identify patients without significant stenosis at the carotid bifurcation, thereby reducing the need for invasive angiography.

Invasive methods

CT angiography

CT angiography is a new technique that can be applied to evaluation of carotid artery stenosis. We find this technique potentially promising. In essence, it may finally combine evaluation of the brain, the intracranial and the extracranial vasculature. It requires intravenous injection of 120 cc contrast. The slipring or spiral CT scan is capable of performing 50 consecutive rotations in 50 s. The thickness of the sections is 3 min. There is continuous overlap and sections are reconstructed at every 1 mm Data acquisition is about 40 s. It takes 15 min for the scanner to reconstruct the images. A three-dimensional reconstruction is then made at an independent workstation. This is partly done by hand and takes between 30 and 45 min. Images of all extra and intracranial major vessels can be obtained. We compared the CT images of 50 carotid bifurcations to standard angiography. Both modalities were in agreement in 41 cases (82 %). The kappa value was 0.85. CTA depicted additional abnormalities as loops, aneurysms and ulcers. A similar study by Schwartz showed agreement in 92 % of cases with a kappa value of 0.9. These values compare favorably to those of MRA. An additional advantage of CTA is the lower failure rate because the patient has to remain motionless for less than a minute. Its major disadvantage is the use of contrast material. Further clinical studies are needed before the definite place of this technique will be established, but we expect that it will reduce the need for conventional arteriography or intraartial DSA.

Angiography

Angiography is the standard diagnostic technique that provides detailed information about the degree of stenosis at the bifurcation and about the degree of irregularity which reflects the presence of ulceration. Angiography delineates not only the bifurcation but also the aortic arch vessels, the distal extracranial carotid and the intracranial vessels. Although rare, anatomic variations are also depicted. Intracranial lesions encompass syphon stenosis, aneurysms, tumors and arteriovenous malformations. Syphon stenosis is present in 6 %, aneurysm in 2 %, tumors in 0.1 % and aortic arch pathology in 0.6 %. The question remains how relevant these lesions are for the decision to perform endarterectomy or not. It is fair to assume that the recent stroke rate is less because of the use of intra-arterial DSA and nonionic contrast media. A final disadvantage of angiography is that it is not as objective as it looks; there is great intra- and interobserver variability, equalling that of duplexscanning.

The presence of intracranial stenosis does not lead to worse results of carotid end-arterectomy and should therefore not be seen as a reason to withhold patients from the benefits of this operation. There may have an influence on long-term prognosis but this is similarly true for patients treated conservatively.

A major advantage of angiography is that it provides a hard copy of the lesion and an anatomical guideline that helps the surgeon to perform the operation well. Finally, angiography is the best diagnostic technique to determine whether a carotid is occluded or not, although it is not infallible. The final argument in favor of angiography is that it is the procedure on which the proof for the beneficial effect of carotid endarterectomy has been based. Other techniques may be as valuable but there is no clinical proof for this assumption and we have to be careful to stay on solid ground regarding this decision making.

Angiography causes discomfort and has risks and costs. Although it may be done as an outpatient procedure, most patients will be hospitalized

Which methods should we use today?

The answer to this question depends to a certain degree on the local expertise with and availability of various techniques. Conventional arteriography or intraarterial DSA are the standard on which the decision to operate or not should generally be made. There is sufficient evidence that angiography is not necessary for all patients with hemispheric cerebrovascular symptoms. Duplexscanning can be used to rule out the presence of significant carotid disease. One has to be careful with proceeding to operation just on the duplexscan outcome. Major prerequisites for such a policy are documented quality assurance in the vascular laboratory and continuous evaluation of mistakes made in those patients in whom arteriography was also used. The technician who performed the test must have no doubt about the severity of the lesion and the surgeon must have sufficient expertise to confirm this while reviewing the duplex personally. The presence of proximal disease, disease continuing distally to the carotid bulb, kinks and coils are reasons to proceed to angiography, before carotid endarterectomy. The possible benefits of carotid endarterectomy without angiography are avoidance of the risk of neurologic complication associated with cerebral angiography, avoidance of discomfort to the patient and a cost saving to the health care system. Surgeons who advocate this approach recommend that it be done only in selected cases. The accuracy of duplex ultrasonography must be known and must be high enough to make this approach reasonable. The patient should have hemispheric symptoms and a hemodynamically, significant carotid artery stenosis appropriate for the lesion. Some surgeons would also recommend computed tomography to exclude intracranial aneurysm or neoplasm and transcranial Doppler ultrasonography to exclude severe intracranial stenosis.

Operation is indicated in patients with 70 % stenosis or more, as measured on angiography. There is a tendency to do the operation without angiography because other techniques such as ultrasound and MR may give the same classification without the inherent risks of angiography and at lower costs. One has to realize however that today's standard practice is to include angiography.

My personal opinion is that I still prefer confirmation of the duplex result by another test before proceeding to surgery. When there is a contraindication to angiography, I do not hesitate to do the operation without it. MRA and CTA are promising but cannot yet be recommended in general for clinical decision making on a large scale. Further clinical studies are required. However, one may savely assume that the days of conventional angiography are coming to an end.

Author's address:
Dimitrios Velecheris, MD
Chief of IKA Hospital
42, Saphous St.,
17676 Kalithea – Athens, Greece

Color-coded duplex ultrasonography of the carotid bifurcation: clinical application in preoperative diagnosis

B. Schulte, D. Beyer

Department of Diagnostic and Interventional Radiology, Krankenhaus Porz am Rhein, Academic Teaching Hospital of the University of Cologne, Germany

For most vascular surgeons and radiologists carotid angiography (conventional angiography and intravenous or intraarterial DSA) is the gold standard to evaluate atherosclerotic stenosis of the carotid bifurcation. For a long time this was commonly accepted in everyday clinical work. However, angiography is still an invasive and furthermore expensive test. Therefore efforts have been made to develop less expensive and less invasive imaging techniques.

Numerous studies have evaluated the ability of ultrasonography to assess the degree of carotid stenosis accurately (1–13).

First, continous wave Doppler provided reliable diagnostic information using two seperate transducers, one to send and one to receive the Doppler signal. To quantify the degree of stenosis it is necessary to assess the peak frequency shift detected in the vessel. Besides the continously audible Doppler sound a Doppler waveform analysis is to be performed which reflects the severity of stenosis. The peak velocity, degree of spatial broadening and internal/common carotid peak velocity ratios were used to determine the percentage of stenosis (1). This technique is best for stenoses greater than 50 %, as carotid stenoses usually begin to produce frequency changes when they exceed 50 % of the vessel diameter.

High-resolution B-mode real-time sonography enables a thorough gray-scale evaluation of extracranial carotid vessels. Imaging in both transverse and longitudinal planes establishes the optimal orientation. Thus it becomes possible to detect small nonstenotic (< 50 %) plaques and to describe their echo morphology.

Later, duplex carotid sonography was introduced as a means of combining high-resolution real-time sonography and pulsed Doppler ultrasound (3). B-mode imaging allows to document the location and to position the Doppler probe by using an accurate scan angle. The recently introduced color-Doppler-flow imaging offers velocity information superimposed on a gray scale ultrasonography image (2, 4, 5, 9). The partial and temporal distribution of color-coded Doppler signal is visualized and the site of maximal stenosis can be detected easily.

Image acquisition in color Doppler ultrasonography

In the 19th century, Johann Doppler first described the Doppler phenomenon as an explanation for color shift in light spectra emitted from stars. The Doppler shift can be described as the change in pitch that results from the relative motion between a source and an observer. In clinical application a fixed source within the transducer is used to apply sound to blood flow and subsequently the change in pitch of reflected sound is measured. Returning echoes are analyzed for amplitude, phase and frequency shift. Amplitude data provide a gray-scale or tissue image (14). As an indicator of blood flow the registered phase and frequency shift is shown as a color assignment superimposed on the standard gray-scale image. The direction of blood flow relative to the Doppler transducer and color box determines the color assignment. Flow toward the transducer will be red and flow away from transducer will be blue. If the vessel is parallel to the Doppler beam no frequency shift will be detected and subsequently no color will be displayed. Finally, color assignment (red or blue) is arbitrary and can be changed in most cases by software configuration.

Studies must be performed with optimal color gain and flow sensitivity setting. The system should be adjusted such that color fills the entire vessel lumen, but does not spill over the adjacent soft tissue. To obtain images of best diagnostic value it is necessary to perform angle correction to maintain the direction of ultrasound beam at approximately 45 to 60 degrees relative to the artery being examined. Further the pulse-repetition frequency can be set to various shift values (kilohertz) depending on actual blood flow velocity anticipated in the given vessel. By adapting the pulse-repetition frequency the frame rate will also be changed. Moreover, different threshold settings are available to perform "slow-flow examinations". These settings are useful if one is searching for a trickle of flow in a preocclusive high-graded carotid artery lesion (4, 12).

Color saturation on the image received, is directly dependent on flow velocity and the angle of sound beam in relation to the longitudinal axis of the flow lumen. High-frequency shifts result in greater color saturation toward the lighter shades of red and blue (4, 5, 9–12).

Furthermore, the color Doppler equipment is capable of performing conventional pulsed Doppler spectral analysis and providing an audible presentation of Doppler signals (3). For most studies this capability is not used in routine examination.

Studies of the extracranial carotid arteries are to be performed with a 5 or 7.5 MHz transducer. The patient is positioned as for a conventional Doppler study. Each examination should include longitudinal and transversal views of the carotid bifurcation obtained from an anterior to posterolateral approach. Imaging quality depends largely on the experience of the examiner. Finally, there will be only a low number of unsatisfactory results. The main reasons for poor imaging quality are a high location of the bifurcation, the inability to hyperextend the neck or a very deeply located carotid system.

Results in clinical application

Color-coded ultrasonography is useful in the evaluation of hemodynamic changes associated with the earliest aspects of atherosclerotic disease.

The examinations are evaluated by observing the degree of luminal narrowing as evidenced by the width of color flow pattern at its narrowest portion relative to the size of the vessel.

Normal carotid arteries show a laminar blood flow which may be interrupted by a transient flow reversal at the origin of the internal carotid artery. This transient flow separation appears at either early or peak systole and may persist for a variable amount of time into the diastole (7, 8).

Color Doppler ultrasonography depicts stenoses by both abnormal color changes and the visible narrowing of the lumen. Thus subtle irregularities of the vessel wall and hypoechoic plaques are better depicted in color-coded ultrasonography than in gray-scale imaging only. In the same way ulcerations and dissections are also better seen in color imaging.

In cases of *low-grade carotid stenosis (40–60 %)* color fading occurs only during systole within a segment of increased flow velocity. There is minimal poststenotic turbulence and in B-mode imaging only minor plaque extent is to be seen.

A *medium-grade carotid stenosis (60–80 %)* shows color fading more circumscribed with increased diastolic flow velocity and turbulent, reversed poststenotic flow. B-mode imaging shows a moderate lumen narrowing.

A *high-grade carotid stenosis (80–90 %)* reveals a segment of marked color fading and severe poststenotic flow reversal and mixed turbulence. Furthermore, there is a reduced prestenotic flow velocity in the common carotid artery. B-mode imaging depicts a severe lumen narrowing (6, 9). In cases of occlusion no color signal will be detected.

In routine examination a quick longitudinal and transversal color Doppler survey is sufficient to pinpoint areas of abnormal flow and heterogeneous color patterns and luminal narrowing. To quantify the point of maximal stenosis, it is possible to measure the peak systolic velocity within the point as maximal mean velocity, as seen on the color image. Percentage of stenosis can generally easily be calculated by directly measuring the flow lumen and then comparing it with the diameter of the vessel itself.

If calcified plaques are encountered associated shadowing precludes to determine luminal narrowing precisely. However, it is sometimes useful to obtain a more posterior or anterior approach without associated shadowing from plaques.

In comparison to conventional gray-scale ultrasonography, color Doppler provides several advantages (1, 9). By the simultaneous two-dimensional display of tissue structure and flow velocity profile the evaluation of the extent of carotid plaque is improved.

Anechoic plaque components that have not be seen in conventional B-mode imaging can be visualized in color Doppler mode by sparing the color flow signal in the absence of any tissue reflection. The differentiation of smooth and irregular surface structures and the identification of ulcerative niches is also improved by color Doppler imaging. This is of major clinical importance as numerous cerebrovascular events are suspected to be of embolic origin due to carotid artery ulcers (10).

Color imaging is especially helpful if there is tortuosity of the vessels because the flow is easier to detect in color than the lumen of the vessel in real-time scanning.

Compared with standard Doppler sonography, color flow scanning has two major advantages. First, it is easier to identify the region of bifurcation and to differentiate internal and external carotid artery by flow detection in branches of the external carotid. Second, if the stenosis is very high-grade only a very narrow trickle of blood may be seen through the stenotic segment. This may be missed more easily conventional Doppler (1, 4, 10).

In comparison with angiography, color-coded Doppler imaging is more accurate in classifying various grades of stenosis. A disadvantage of angiography is that the arterial wall remains invisible and therefore the degree of luminal narrowing is more difficult to be estimated (13).

Conclusions

Color flow vascular imaging represents a significant advance in Doppler imaging technology. It shows to be an accurate method for depicting atherosclerotic plaque and for quantifying the percentage of stenosis including velocity measurements.

The results concerning location and grade of carotid stenosis are more reliable than those obtained by conventional Doppler, B-mode imaging or angiography.

References

1. Carroll BA (1991) Carotid Sonography. Radiology 178: 303–313
2. Erickson SJ, Mewissen MW, Foley WD, Lawson TL, Middleton WD, Quiroz FA, Macrander SJ, Lipchik EO (1989) Stenosis of Internal Carotid Artery: Assessment Using Color Doppler Imaging Compered with Angiography. AJR 152: 1299–1305
3. Hallam MJ, Reid JM, Cooperberg PL (1989) Color Flow Doppler and Conventional Duplex Scanning of the Carotid Bifurcation: Prospective, Double-blind, Correative Study. AJR 152: 1101–1105
4. Hetzel A, Eckenweber B, Trummer B, Wernz M, von Reutern GM (1993) Farbkodierte Duplexsonographie bei präokklusiven Stenosen der Arteria carotis interna. Ultraschall in Med, 14: 240–246
5. Hübsch von P, Schwaighofer B, Karnel F, Braunsteiner A, Frühwald F, Pichler W, Trattnig S (1988) Farbkodierte Dopplersonographie der Karotiden. Fortschr Röntgenstr 149: 189–192
6. Jacobs NM, Grant EG, Schellinger D, Byrd MC, Richardson JD, Cohan SL (1985) Duplex Carotid Sonography: Criteria for Stenosis, Accuracy and Pitfalls. Radiology: 154: 385–391
7. Middleton WD, Foley WD, Lawson TL (1988) Flow Reversal in the Normal Carotid Bifurcation: Color Doppler Flow Imaging Analysis. Radiology 167: 207–210
8. Middleton WD, Foley WD, Lawson TL (1988) Color-Flow Doppler Imaging of Carotid Artery Abnormalities. AJR 150: 419–425
9. Polak JF, Dobkin GR, O'Leary DH, Wang AM, Cutler SS (1989) Internal Carotid Artery Stenosis: Accuracy and Reproducibility of Color-Doppler-assisted Duplex Imaging. Radiology 173: 793–798
10. Steinke W, Kloetzsch C, Hennerici M (1990) Carotid Artery Disease Assessed by Color Doppler Flow Imaging: Correlation with Standard Doppler Sonography and Angiography. AJNR 11: 259–266
11. Trattnig von S, Pölzleitner D, Hübsch P, Daha K, Matula Ch, Magometschnigg H (1992) Nicht-invasive Verlaufskontrolle mittels farbkodierter Doppler-Sonographie nach operativen Eingriffen an den extrakraniellen hirnversorgenden Arterien. Fortschr Röntgenstr 156,3: 224–227
12. Trattnig von S, Hübsch P, Barton P, Karnel F, Sautner Th, Schwaighofer B, Kretschmer G (1991) Durchgängigkeit der Carotis externa und interna bei Patienten mit Carotis-communis-Okklusion: Nachweis in der farbkodierten Doppler Sonographie. Fortschr Röntgenstr 154,1: 44–48
13. Tschammler von A, Landwehr P, Höhmann M, Moll R, Wittenberg G, Lackner K (1991) Farbkodierte Duplexsonographie der extrakraniellen hirnversorgenden Arterien: diagnostische Aussagekraft und Fehlerquellen im Vergleich zu i.a. DSA. Fortschr Röntgenstr 155,5: 452–459
14. Wolf KJ, Fobbe F (1993) Farbkodierte Duplexsonographie. Grundlagen und klinische Anwendung. Georg Thieme Verlag, Stuttgart New-York

Author's address:
Bernhard Schulte, MD
Department of Radiology
Acad. Teach.-Hospital Porz, Univ. of Cologne
Urbacher Weg 19
51149 Köln, Germany

Ultrasonic and histopathological characteristics of the carotid plaque

A. Katsamouris

Department of Vascular Surgery, Iraklio University Hospital, Iraklio, Greece

The risk of stroke has been associated with progression of atherosclerotic disease at the carotid artery bifurcation (2, 3, 12, 15). In this regard, features related to surface and composition characteristics of the atherosclerotic plaque, such as ulceration and intraplaque hemorrhage, are thought to be of a great pathogenetic importance. Therefore, detection of plaque components that could be the harbingers of future stroke is of critical concern (7, 8, 9, 11, 13, 22).

B-mode sonography, aided by color flow imaging, has been recognized as the most accurate noninvasive method for assessment of atherosclerosis at carotid artery bifurcation (23). High resolution B-mode sonography offers excellent visualization of the carotid plaque, but its ability to identify plaque characteristics most likely related to cerebrovascular ischaemic attacks remains in question (14, 20, 23).

In this presentation, based on our relative study performed in 40 patients with symptomatic and asymptomatic casotid plaque, we discuss the reliability of carotid plaque ultrasonography in depicting plaque pathology, thus providing clinically relevant plaque classification.

Clearly, there is a need to diagnose potential stroke-producing plaques so that carotid endarterectomy can be undertaken when appropriate and avoided when unnecessary. The results of the European Carotid Endarterectomy Trial in symptomatic patients with an internal carotid artery stenosis more than 70 % have shown that at 3 years after presentation of symptoms and treatment, the total risk of surgical mortality and stroke was 12.3 % in patients after endarterectomy and 21.9 % in medically treated patients (3). Therefore, a subgroup of patients may exist among those having an internal carotid artery stenosis more than 70 % that is at a high risk to develop major ischemic neurological events.

Our study has shown that, for an internal carotid artery stenosis greater than 70 %, the severity of clinical presentation was strongly related to the degenerative changes ocurring in the plaque. The predominant constituent of the plaques, whether symptomatic or not, consisted of fibrous tissue. However, plaques containing less than 60 % fibrous tissue ("soft" plaques), were highly related to the development of stroke, while those containing more than 60 % fibrous tissue ("hard" plaques), were mostly found in patients presenting with T.I.A. or without symptoms. The differences in respect to plaque soft tissue component were also significant: the plaques of the patients presenting with stroke contained significantly more soft tissue (33 ± 9 %) than those of the patients presenting with the T.I.A. (17 ± 9 %) or without symptoms (14 ± 4 %). Other quantitative and/or qualitative studies have also shown that plaque composition may play a more important role in the pathogenesis of cerebral ischemic episodes than the degree of internal carotid artery stenosis *per se*.

Thus, Seeger and Klingman have demonstrated that the plaques from patients with neurological symptoms contain significantly more total lipid and cholesterol, and less collagen from those of asymptomatic patients (19). Similarly, Lean et al. have shown a predominance of plaque non-fibrous component mixed with cholersterol in symptomatic as compared with asymptomatic patients (10). Parallel to these pathological studies, Reilly et al. have indicated a poor correlation between luminal stenosis and clinical status of patients, since no high-grade stenotic lesions were identified in their stroke patients (17).

In our series, plaque hemorrhage and ulceration were equally distributed among our patients and were not related to their clinical status. Furthermore, plaque content of hemorrhage was not significantly different among asymptomatic patients or those presenting with stroke or T.I.A. This is at variance with most other studies that stressed the importance of plaque hemorrhage in the development of cerebrovascular events, reporting plaque hemorrhage in up to 80 % of symptomatic patients (6, 7, 11, 13). However, in these studies plaque composition was not analyzed. In our study carotid plaque histology was undertaken objectively by identifying and quantifying the plaque components and expressing them as percentage of the total plaque content. In our opinion, the methodology allowed us to asses plaque composition more accurately and to compare it with the clinical status and ultrasonographic data more adequately.

In agreement with our findings, recent studies conducted in a similar way demonstrated that hemorrhage and ulceration were not the dominant plaque characteristics in symptomatic patients (1, 10, 21). More recently, Feeley et al. found that hemorrhage constituted 2 % and 1 % of asymptomatic and symptomatic plaques, respectively (14). They maintained that the predominance of nonfibrous constituent was a pink amorphous material mixed with cholesterol, which comprised 7 % of asymptomatic and 27 % of symptomatic plaques. Most probably, this pink amorphous material/cholesterol component has been designated as hemorrhage by other authors. However, similar to our findings, Feeley et al. were unable to identify any blood breakdown with standard histologic stains or immunoperoxidase staining techniques with antifactor VIII and antihuman platelet glycoprotein IIIa antibodies (4, 10). Additionally, Bassiouny et al. did not classify this pink amorphous material as hemorrhage, but refer to it as plaque necrosis, including atheromatous debris and cholesterol clefts (1).

At present, atherosclerosis is a complex disease process that is not completely understood (18). The data of our study support the hypothesis that "soft" plaques appears to play an important role in the pathogenesis of cerebrovascular events. We postulate that under suitable hemodynamic and metabolic conditions (1, 18), the unstable plaque component of soft tissue may be disrupted leading to stroke by discharging its content or by stimulating thrombogenesis. Therefore, plaque composition could be a useful discriminating factor in selecting asymptomatic patients for either carotid endarterectomy or conservative treatment.

B-mode sonography, aided by color flow imaging, has gained worldwide acceptance as the noninvasive method of choice for assessing atherosclerotic disease at the carotid artery bifurcation (23, 24). However, some ambiguity still exists regarding the uniformity in interpreting and reporting the features of ultrasonic plaque "biopsy" (23). Most of the descriptive terms used have a rather broad character. Thus, determination of plaque composition has been attempted by describing lesion echogenecity, such as hypoechoic, hyperechoic, and isoechoic. Plaque complications such as surface fibrous cap fracture, ulceration, and hemorrhage have been assessed in terms of surface regularity or irregularity, and plaque ulceration or defect. Finally, the overall internal echo pattern of the plaque has been characterized either homogeneous (uniform) or heterogeneous (nonuniform). In our opinion this ambiguity may be explained by the fact that studies comparing ultrasonic plaque as characteristics and plaque composition have been focused, with rare exceptions (4), on qualitative changes of the plaque only, such as the presence or absence of hemorrhage or ulceration. No attempt was made to assess the compatibility between ultrasonic plaque features and the various plaque constituents based on quantitative measurements.

Pathologic accumulation of soft tissue, collagen or calcium deeply modify the acoustical fingerprints of the normal tissue. Thus, plaque soft tissue, including hemorrhage, and qualitative changes of plaque stroma, such as loose stroma, are mainly featuring as echolucent or hypoechoic areas, while plaque dense fibrous tissue is responsible for the echodence plaque character (4, 16, 17, 19). The hypothesis under consideration is that a particular plaque component might determine a specific ultrasound-tissue interaction, ultimately detectable through the analysis of the acquired ultrasonic imaging.

In our study, we used as a criterion both qualitative and quantitative changes identified in the plaque pathology, so as to comparatively test the validity of all major descriptive terms in use for ultrasonic characterization of the plaque. In agreement with previously reported results (4, 14), our findings clearly showed that plaque surface regularity, irregularity, ulceration and plaque hemorrhage were inconsistent with plaque pathology. Most of the above ultrasonic features were visualized similarly as small or large echolucent areas, mainly reflecting the soft tissue component of the plaque and/or qualitative changes of the plaque stroma, thus being insufficient to identify plaque ulceration or hemorrhage.

Comparable results were reported by others, as well (4, 14). In a most recent report, the Committee on Standards in Noninvasive Vascular Testing has recommended that characterization of plaque morphology "should be confined to whether the plaque is homogeneous or heterogeneous", recognizing that further research may produce a more comprehensive and clinically appropriate classification (23). In the classification followed in the our study, plaque Types 1 and 4 were both homogeneous, but the homogeneously echogenic plaque Type 1 consisted of considerably more fibrous tissue than the homogeneously echolucent plaque Type 4 (78 ± 6 % vs 58 ± 13 %, respectively). Furthermore, it was the echogenic (plaque Types A and B) and not the heterogenic character of the plaque (plaque Types 2 and 3) that was better associated with plaque pathology.

Additionally, it appears that the classification of the plaques according to their echogenicity provides more clinically relevant information of atherosclerotic disease. In our series, the association between the plaque type and clinical presentation showed that there was a predominance of echolucent plaques (plaque Type B) in the symptomatic and of echogenic plaques (plaque Type A) in the asymptomatic patients. These results are comparable with those reported by other authors who used similar plaque type classification. Thus, Steffen et al. (1989), reported that in symptomatic patients the echolucent plaques were more common (67 %), whereas in asympomatic patients the most commonly encountered plaques (86 %) were echogenic (20). More recently, Geroulakos et al. (1993), investigating the ultrasonic plaque characteristics in a population similar to ours, found that the echolucent plaques predominated in symptomatic patients, concluding that this plaque type is unstable and tends to embolize (5). Furthermore, and in agreement with our findings, the distribution of the heterogeneous plaques among their symptomatic and asymptomatic patients was less consistent as compared with the echogenic plaque Type A and echolucent plaque Type B.

In the light of the above, it is suggested that plaques containing greater than 60 % fibrous tissue seem not as likely to be associated with severe cerebrovascular events as plaques with lower amounts of fibrous tissue. Characterization of plaques in regard to their echogenicity, as mainly echogenic (Type A) or mainly echolucent (Type B), appears to be a comprehensive and clinically appropriate classification, since the echogenic character of the plaque is better associated with plaque pathology and clinical presentation. Adoption of the suggested ultrasonographic plaque classification might prove useful in studying the natural history of asymptomatic patients with a high-grade carotid plaque stenosis and in identifying a high-risk subgroup that might benefit from surgical treatment.

References

1. Bassiouny HS, Davis H, Massawa N, Gewerts BL, Glagov S, Zarins CK (1989) Critical carotid stenosis: morpholigical and chemical similarity between symptomatic and asymptomatic plaques. J Vasc Surg 9: 202–212
2. Chambers BR, Norris JW (1986) Outcome in patients with asymptomatic neck bruits. N Engl J Med 315: 860–865
3. European Carotid Surgery Trialists' Collaborative group (1991) MRC European Carotid Surgery Trial: interim results for symptomatic patients with severe (70–99 %) or with mild (0–29 %) carotid stenosis. Lancet 337: 1235–1243
4. Feeley TM, Leen EJ, Colgan MP, Moore DJ, Hourihane DO, Shanik GD (1991) Histologic characteristics of carotid artery plaque. J Vasc Surg 13: 719–724
5. Geroulakos G, Ramaswami G, Nicolaides A et al. (1993) Characterization of symptomatic and asymptomatic carotid plaques using high-resolution real-time ultrasonography. Br J Surg 80: 1274–1277
6. Imparato AM, Riles TS, Gorstein F (1979) The carotid bifurcation plaque: pathologic findings associated with cerebral ischaemia. Stroke 10: 238–245
7. Imparato AM, Riles TS, Mintzer R, Baumann FG (1983) The importance of hemorrhage in the relationship between gross morphologic characteristics and cerebral symptoms in 376 carotid artery plaques. Ann Surg 97: 195–203
8. Langsfield M, Grav-Weale AC, Lushy RJ (1989) The role of plaque morphology and diameter reduction in the development of new symptoms in asymptomatic carotid arteries. J Vasc Surg 9: 548–557
9. Leahy AL, McCollum PT, Feeley TM et al. (1988) Duplex ultrasonography and selection of patients for carotid endarterectomy: plaque morphology or luminal narrowing. J Vasc Surg 8: 558–562
10. Leen EJ, Feeley TM, Colgan MP et al. (1990) "Haemorrhagic" carotid plaque does not contain haemorrhage. Eur J Vasc Surg 4: 123–128
11. Lusby RJ, Ferrell LD, Ehrenfeld WK, Stoney RJ, Wylie EJ (1982) Carotid plaque hemorrhage: its role in production of cerebral ischaemia. Arch Surg 117: 1479–1488
12. North American Symptomatic Carotid Endarterectomy Trial Collaborators (1991) Beneficial effect of carotid endarterectomy in symptomatic patients with high-grade stenosis. N Engl J Med 325: 445–453
13. O'Donnell TF, Erdoes L, Mackey WC et al. (1985) Correlation of B-mode ultrasound imaging and arteriography with pathologic findings at carotid endarterectomy. Arch Surg 120: 443–449
14. O'Learly DH, Holen J, Ricotta JJ, Roes S, Schenk EA (1987) Carotid bifurcation disease: prediction of ulceration with B-Mode US. Radiology 162: 523–525
15. Pessin MS, Duncan GW, Mohr JP, Poskanzer DC (1977) Clinical and angiographic features of carotid transient ischemic attacks. N Engl J Med 296: 358–362
16. Picano E, Landini L, Lattanzi F et al. (1988) Ultrasonic tissue characterization of atherosclerosis: state of the art 1988. J Nucl Med Allied Sci 32: 174–185
17. Reilly LR, Lusby RJ, Hughes L, Ferrell LD, Stoney RJ, Ehrenfeld WK (1983) Carotid plaque histology using real time ultrasonography: clinical and therapeutic implications. Am J Surg 146: 188–193
18. Ross R (1993) The pathogenesis of atherosclerosis: a perspective for the 1990s. Nature 362: 801–809
19. Seeger J, Klingman N (1987) The relationship between carotid plaque composition and neurological symptoms. J Surg Res 43: 78–85
20. Steffen CM, Gray-Wealle AC, Byrne KE, Hayes SJ, Lusby RJ (1989) Carotid atheroma: ultrasound appearance in symptomatic and asymptomatic vessels. Aust N Z J Surg 59: 529–534
21. Svindland A, Torvic A (1988) Atherosclerotic carotid disease in asymptomatic individuals: an histologic study of 53 cases. Acta Neurol Scand 78: 506–517
22. Thiele BL, Young JV, Chikos PM, Hirsch JM, Strandness DE Jr (1980) Correlation of arteriographic findings and symptoms on cerebrovascular disease. Neurology 30: 1041–1046
23. Thiele BL, Jones AM, Hobson RW et al. (1992) Standards in noninvasive vascular testing of the Joint Council of the Society for Vascular Surgery and the North American Chapter of the International Society for Cardiovascular Surgery. J Vasc Surg 15: 495–503
24. Tsuruda JS, Saloner D, Anderson C (1991) Noninvasive evaluation of cerebral ischaemia: trends for the 1990s. Circulation 83 (suppl I): I-176–I-189

Author's address:
Prof. A. Katsamouris, MD, PhD
Chief of Vascular Surgery
Iraklio University Hospital
Vouton & Stavrakion
71100 Iraklio-Crete, Greece

Magnetic resonance angiography (MRA) of the carotid and vertebral arteries

G. Wedekind, D. Beyer

Department of Diagnostic and Interventional Radiology, Krankenhaus Porz am Rhein, Academic Teaching Hospital of the University of Cologne, Germany

Cerebrovascular disease is the third leading cause of death in Western Europe. Cerebral ischemic disease caused by atherosclerotic carotid artery disease is responsible for a considerable number of strokes (9, 15).

Conventional cerebral angiography and color-coded Doppler ultrasonography are currently the accepted preoperative tests to determine if a significant carotid or vertebral stenosis or other pathologies of the carotid bifurcation requiring surgical intervention are present.

The excellent visualization of the carotid and vertebral arteries by magnetic resonance angiography (MRA) suggests its usefullness in the evaluation of vessel stenoses in patients with cerebral ischemia or infarction (7).

The increasing availability and improvements in software and hardware, especially on 0.5 Tesla MR-units, makes MRA more and more competitive to other angiographic techniques (19, 22).

With the introduction of the so-called time-of-flight techniques in MRA, this method became a serious alternative to conventional tests (3, 6, 20).

MRA has several obvious advantages over conventional angiography. It is a safe, rapid and noninvasive technique allowing many projections of the examined vessels, due to a wide range of postprocessing options (10, 25). The use of contrast agents is not necessary (15).

MRA consists of a physiological study of moving blood, using a complex interaction between the physical characteristics of blood flow and the MR-pulse sequence, to depict a visible signal within the vessel producing an angiogramlike image (3).

If normal flow within a normal non stenotic-vessel is examined, the detected signal gives an exact impression of the perfused lumen. Vessels with stenoses, aneurysms, kinkings, coilings or other irregularities do not show normal laminar flow. Artifactual loss of signal may often lead to an overestimation of the stenosis (5).

The purpose of our study was to determine the efficacy of 2-D time-of-flight MRA in characterizing pathologies of the carotid bifurcation and vertebral arteries by using conventional angiography and color-coded Doppler ultrasonography as the standard of reference.

Materials and methods

Between March and August 1994, 124 carotid bifurcations and 124 vertebral arteries in 62 consecutive patients (42 males, 20 females), with neurologic symptoms of hemispheric ischemia and/or unilateral or bilateral stenosis of the internal carotid arteries depicted by ultrasonography and color-coded Doppler, underwent 2D-TOF MRA and DSA. Two patients did not complete the MR-angiographic examinations due to claustrophobia. The oldest patient was 87 years old, the youngest 45 years old. The median age was 65.8 years.

All patients were examined with a 0.5 Tesla superconducting imaging system (MRT-50 A-Super, Toshiba Medical Systems, Japan) by using an optimized 2D TOF sequence (16).

By applying a conventional routine linear polarized neck coil, a sagittal localizer was used to plan the axial oblique directed sections.

To avoid motion and swallowing artifacts we used a conventional cervical collar of foam rubber, normally applied in traumatology, to stabilize the patients neck in the coil and to avoid swallowing, which was proved to be effective.

A 2D TOF-angiography aquisition with 58–72 slices (thickness 3.5 mm, 1 mm overlap) was performed with a so-called "walking saturation band" and 35/11 (repetition time msec/echo time ms). The duration of this sequence was 9–13 min dependent on the number of slices applied. The whole examination took about 25 min.

Postprocessing subvolumes were generated to isolate each side of supraaortal arteries creating 18 maximum-intensity-projection (MIP) images at 10-degree increments around the body axis, starting from a line between the ICA and the ECA. The size of the region of interest (ROI) needed was individual depending on the spatial extension of the vessels.

None of the examinations was repeated when motion was present, and none of the patients received a sedative premedication.

When motion affected one or several sections, which were seen clearly to be out of alignment, but did not interfere with evaluation of stenosis, the examination was graded as "motion present" but still diagnostic.

All intravenous DSA examinations were performed with a cubital vein approach. DSA was unsuitable in five patients due to a severe contrast agent reaction in the past despite administration of cortisone and antihistamine, or untreated hyperthyreosis. DSA imaging was performed in anterior-posterior and lateral-oblique projections.

The DSA angiagrams and MR angiograms and original 2D axial slices were reviewed blinded to the patient's name and clinical history. The presence of additional clinically significant lesions, including arterial occlusions, kinking coiling and aneurysms were recorded.

The evaluation of stenoses was performed by assessment of the stenosis relative to the normal segment of the arteries proximal and distal to the stenosis (none = 0 %, minor = 1–15 %, moderate = 16–49 %, severe = 50–70 %, high grade = 70–90 %, filiform > 90 %) (1).

Results

Only one MRA examination was graded "un-diagnostic". About 30 % had motion artifacts but were still evaluatable.

In comparison to the DSA examinations the 2D TOF technique had excellent results in depicting minor, moderate or severe stenosis. In a few cases, MRA was superior to DSA due to the postprocessing capabilities of MIP. Thus overprojection of vessels (ICA, ECA) as sometimes occurs with DSA is avoided. MRA is the only diagnostic method able to depict the carotid bifurcation without any interfering projection effects, even with anatomic variations. The evaluation of high grade or filiform stenosis did not create problems if an endarterectomy was indicated or not. The only inaccuracy was the exact estimation of vessel narrowing between 80 and over 90 %. A distinction between a long high-grade stenosis and a short filiform stenosis was not possible with MRA. Due to turbulent flow in the poststenotic part of the vessel, signal voids appear. Recurrence to laminar flow with normal signal depends on the length and/or the grade of the stenosis (5, 13, 15, 21).

Elongations, kinkings and coilings of vessels could be depicted excellently as well. But we had problems in evaluation of the horizontal course of these elongated vessels. Signal void in these areas occurred and we could not decide between vessel narrowing and normal flow. The evaluation in patients with circular atherosclerotic plaques was definitely superior to color-coded Doppler ultrasonography and DSA. MRA did not show any artifacts when calcified plaques were present.

In one patient we saw an aneurysm of the ICA. The diameter of the perfused lumen was determined from the MIP images and axial sections as well. Due to the turbulent flow within the aneurysm the signal given by moving spins is less than that from laminar flow of other liquids.

In another patient at first we diagnosed an occlusion of the left vertebral artery because of missing signal within the vessel. DSA examination showed a retrograde flow as a sign of subclavian steal syndrome. When subclavian steal is clinically suspected and has to be differentiated from occlusion a second data aquisition with an inverse scan direction becomes necessary.

Discussion

2D Time-of-Flight MRA of the carotid bifurcation and the vertebral arteries at 0.5 T is able to show in an excellent manner the whole range of pathologic variations (14, 21). It consists of a semiquantitative method for evaluating vessel narrowing, without the use of contrast agents or x-ray. Overestimation of narrowing in the carotid bifurcation, proximal ICA and ECA, due to turbulent flow with consecutive flow void, and/or the so-called "flow separation phenomena" reported by a few authors, did not create diagnostic difficulties (1, 11, 26) even if the subjective appearance of stenoses in MRA images is not transferable to DSA.

The length of a flow void in a stenotic vessel is caused by three factors: degree of stenosis, velocity of blood flow and the length of the atherosclerotic plaque (11, 17, 22, 24). The knowledge of artifacts especially in MIP is essential for the right diagnosis of vessel narrowing (2).

The limiting factor of 2D TOF of the carotid bifurcation is still the small field of view which can be applied because we do not see the aortic arch and the skull base simultaneously (4, 6, 18). Lesions of the proximal carotid artery and the intracranial vessels thus cannot be detected during one examination. But the appearance of alterations in these regions may alter surgical management.

At the moment, real indications for applying MRA of the extracranial vessels are: suspected stenosis of the carotid bifurcation in patients with intolerance of x-ray contrast agents due to renal insufficiency, hyperthyreosis, allergy or severe cardiovascular disease.

The substitution of DSA for examinations of the supraaortal arteries at the moment can only be performed in rare cases by MRA (12). However, there is no doubt about the usefulness of MRA as a supplemental tool in the diagnosis of vessel pathologies, especially in cases of non corresponding preliminary tests. It is noteworthy that MRA as a non-invasive technique in many cases is given greater preference by the patient himself.

With new coil techniques and software improvements hopefully available in the near future, MRA will be able to increasingly substitute DSA.

References

1. Anderson CM, Saloner D, Lee RE (1992) Assessment of carotid artery stenosis by MR angiography: comparison with X-ray angiography and color-coded Doppler ultrasound. AJNR 13: 989–1003
2. Anderson CM, Saloner D, Tsuruda JS (1990) Artifacts in Maximum-Intensity-Projection display of MR angiograms. AJR March 154: 623–629
3. Barr RG (1992) MR vascular imaging of the head and neck. Resonant Ideas Newsletter for Toshiba America Medical Systems, Spring Volume VI No. 1
4. Dillon EH, van Leeuwen MS, Fernandez MA (1993) CT-angiography: Application to the evaluation of carotid artery stenosis. Radiology 189: 211–219
5. Fürst G, Kahn T, Sitzer M (1993) Quantifizierung extrakranieller Karotisstenosen: Magnetresonanz-angiographie und Doppler-Sonographie versus intraarterielle Angiographie. Fortschr Röntgenstr 159,4: 368–374 German art
6. Furura Y, Isoda H, Takahashi M (1992) Magnetic resonance angiography of extracranial carotid and vertebral arteries, including their origins: comparison with DSA. Neuroradiology 35: 42–45
7. Heiserman JE, Drayer BP, Fram EK (1992) Carotid artery stenosis: clinical efficacy of TWO-dimensional Time-of-Flight MR angiography. Radiology 182: 761–768
8. Heinz ER, Yeates AE, Djang WT (1989) Significant extracranial carotid stenosis: detection on routine cerebral MR images. Radiology 170: 843–848
9. Huston J III, Lewis BD, Wiebers DO (1993) Carotid artery: prospective blinded comparison of Two-dimensional Time-of-Flight MR angiography with conventional angiography and Duplex ultrasound. Radiology 186: 339–344
10. Kido DK, Barsotti JB, Rice LZ, Rothenberg BM (1991) Evaluation of carotid artery bifurcation: comparison of magnetic resonance angiography and digital subtraction arch aortography. Neuroradiology 33: 48–51
11. Krug B, Kugel H, Friedmann G (1992) Experimentelle Untersuchungen zur magnetresonanztomographischen und magnetresonanzangiographischen Darstellung poststenotischer Strömungsmuster. Fortschr Röntgenstr 156,5: 475–481 German art
12. Laster RE, Acker JD, Halford HH III (1993) Assessment of MR angiography for evaluation of cervical Carotid bifurcation disease. AJNR 14: 681–688
13. Laub G, Ruggieri P, Felber S (1988) 3D MR angiography of Carotid arteriosclerotic disease. Poster contributed to Second European Congress of NMR in Medicine and Biology June, Berlin
14. Levy C, Laissy JP, Raveau V (1994) Carotid and vertebral artery dissections: three-dimensional Time-of-Flight MR angiography and MR imaging versus conventional angiography. Radiology 190: 97–103
15. Litt AW, Eidelman EM, Pinto RS (1991) Diagnosis of carotid artery stenosis: comparison of 2DFT Time-of-Flight MR angiography with contrast angiography in 50 patients. AJNR 12: 149–154
16. Machida Y, Kitane S, Makita J (1994) Three-dimensional MR angiography of the head and neck. Medical Review for Toshiba Medical Systems No. 37: 1–9
17. Masaryk AM, Ross JS, Di Cello MC (1991) 3DFT MR angiography of the carotid bifurcation: potential and limitations as a screening examination. Radiology 179: 797–804
18. Masaryk TJ, Modic MT, Ruggieri PM (1989) Three-dimensional (volume) gradient-echo-imaging of the carotid bifurcation: preliminary clinical experience. Radiology 171: 801–806
19. Pavone P (1992) Low-field MRA images carotid arteries. Diagnostic Imaging Nov: 211–218
20. Pavone P, Marsili L, Catalano C (1992) Carotid arteries: evaluation with low-field-strength MR-angiographie. Radiology 184: 401–404
21. Polak JF, Kalina P, Donaldson MC (1993) Carotid endarterectomy: preoperative evaluation of candidates with combined Doppler sonography and MR angiography. Radiology 186: 333–338
22. Polak JF, Bajakian RL, O'Leary DO (1992) Detection of internal carotid artery stenosis: comparison of MR angiography, colored Doppler sonography and arteriography. Radiology 182: 35–40
23. Schwartz RB, Jones KM, Chernoff DM (1992) Common carotid artery bifurcation: evaluation with spiral-CT. Radiology 185: 513–519

24. Seiderer M, Kröner KK, Müller E (1988) EKG-getriggerte kernspintomographische Blutflußgeschwindigkeitsmessung in den Karotiden: Vergleich mit Duplex-Sonographie. Digit Bilddiagn 8: 110–114 German art
25. Turnipseed WD, Kennell TW, Turski PA (1994) Magnetic resonance angiography and duplex imaging: noninvasive tests for selecting symptomatic carotid endarterectomy candidates. Radiology 191: 591
26. Wasserman BA, Haacke EM, Li D (1994) Carotid plaque formation and its evaluation with angiography, ultrasound and MR angiography. JMRI 4: 515–527

Author's address:
Gregor Wedekind, MD
Department of Diagnostic and
Interventional Radiology
Acad. Teach.-Hospital Porz, Univ. of Cologne
Urbacher Weg 19
51149 Köln, Germany

Perioperative monitoring during carotid surgery – role of the local anaesthesia

C. Liapis

Athens University Medical School, Greece

Stroke is a problem of enormous magnitude and remains a major cause of disability and death. According to the NIH stroke survey, about 407 000 patients were admitted with new strokes each year in the 1970s in the U.S.A.

Although the incidence of cerebral infarction has declined by almost 50 % in the last 30 years, more than 80 % of the strokes are thromboembolic in origin (1, 2).

Carotid endarterectomy is performed with increased frequency. The current annual figure for the U.S.A. has increased from 15 000 in 1971 to 104 000 in 1984 (3), thus establishing the carotid endarterectomy as the most frequently performed vascular procedure. Similar figures are reported in Europe (4). Despite this popularity, the inherent disadvantage of the operation (i.e., posibility of stroke) both attracts critics and stimulates vascular surgeons to seek a safer way of performing the procedure. This is where the old question arises: to shunt or not to shunt. And despite the use of various methods like continuous EEG monitoring and ICA stump pressure, still the selection of patients to be shunted remains controversial, at least to the surgeons who have not made up their minds to shunt all or to shunt none (5).

The answer to the question for some is very simple. Do the operation with the patient awake (6, 7).

In order to test the validity of this statement the following prospective study was performed.

Materials and methods

From 1984 to 1994, out of 408 carotid endarterectomies, we selected two groups of 50 patients each, operated under general anesthesia (A) or local anesthesia Xylocaine 2 % and light sedation. The age and sex distribution are shown in Table 1.

The mean age was 64 ± 12 for group A and 61 ± 11 for group B. Indications for surgery are shown in Table 2. Most of the patients were operated upon for TIAs (66 % in group A, 70 % in group B).

The patients in group A were operated in the standard fashion, under general halothane anesthesia.

Indwelling shunt was used in 4 % of the cases. The indications are shown in Table 3 and were a ICABP of less than 50 mmHg together with an inadequate back flow and contralateral high grade stenosis.

In group B the patients received light sedation with diazepam and pethidine, with local anesthesia of about 20 cc xylocaine 2 % along the anterior border of the sternocleidomastoid muscle. An additional 2 – 3 cc were needed for the carotid sheath.

The operation then continues in the usual fashion. A shunt was used in 3 (6 %) of the patients because of manifestations of neurologic malfunction appropriate to the operated side under 3 min trial carotid crossclamping.

150 mg of dipyridamole and 250 of aspirin were given daily following surgery in both groups. Antiplatelet therapy was initiated 7 days before surgery. A PTFE patch was used in one case in group B.

The patients were examined clinically postoperatively and before discharge. Neurologic symptoms are referred as temporal deficits if lasting less than 24 h and permanent if lasting for longer period of time. Statistical analysis was done by X^2 test.

Table 1. Age and sex distribution of two groups

Group A	(General Anesthesia)	n = 50
Male	n = 33	(66 %)
Female	n = 17	(34 %)
Age	61 ± 12	
Group B	(Local Anesthesia)	n = 50
Male	n = 37	(74 %)
Female	n = 13	(26 %)
Age	61 ± 11	

Table 2. Indications for Surgery

Group A	(General Anesthesia)	TIAs	33	(66 %)
		Previous Stroke	5	(10 %)
		High Grade Stenosis	12	(24 %)
Group B	(Local Anesthesia)	TIAs	35	(70 %)
		Previous Stroke	4	(8 %)
		High Grade Stenosis	10	(20 %)
		Prophylactic for CABG	1	(2 %)

Table 3. Indications for shunting

Group A (General Anesthesia)	n = 4 (8 %)
ICABP < 50 % Contralateral high grade stenosis Inadequate back flow	
Group B (Local Anesthesia)	n = 3 (6 %)
Manifestation of neurologic Malfunction	

Results

The results are shown in Table 4. In group A we had 4 % neurologic deficits (2 % temporal – 2 % permanent). In group B there was a 6 % neurologic deficit (4 % temporal, 2 % permanent). Mortality rate was 0 % for group A and 2 % for group B.

Temporal cranial nerve injuries were 4 % for group A and 8 % for group B. X^2 test statistical analysis shows a $p > 0.05$ (n.s.). The deficits in both groups developed in all but one case about 6 to 8 h following surgery. The fatal outcome in group B was of a patient with a stroke in evolution. One reoperation was performed in group B when neurologic deficit developed in a patient with a previous stroke following surgery.

No explanation for the stroke was found. Hypertension was noted in 3 (6 %) of the patients in group A and in 5 (10 %) in group B. Motor speech malfunction was noted in 2 (4 %) of group A and 4 (8 %) of group B patients, which was temporary in nature.

The patient acceptance of local anesthesia was excellent in our study and in others (6–9), thus we did not have to convert the procedure to general anesthesia in any of our cases. The routine use of antiplatelet agents did not seem to cause any significant side-effects and no patient required surgery for developing hematoma. It seems that the use of these agents is beneficial following carotid endarterectomy by reducing platelet deposition in the arteriotomy, particularly if a patch has been used (12).

Conclusions

1) The type of anesthesia did not alter the results of the operation in our two groups ($p > 0.05$).

2) Carotid endarterectomy under local is the ideal procedure for surgeons who shunt patients selectively.

Table 4. Results of carotid endarterectomy

Group A (General Anesthesia)	n = 50	
No deficits	48	(96 %)
Temporal deficits	1	(2 %)
Permanent deficits	1	(2 %)
Mortality	0	(0 %)
Cranial nerv injury	4	(8 %)
Group B (Local Anesthesia)	n = 50	
No deficits	477	(94 %)
Temporal deficits	2	(4 %)
Permanent deficits	1	(2 %)
Mortality	1	(2 %)
Cranial nerv injury	4	(8 %)

$p > 0.05$ (x^2-test)

There are, of course, certain disadvantages: a) the surgeon must be adequately fast. One cannot prolong the procedure more than 90 min or the patient becomes restless. b) patients with high carotid bifurcations and short necks could provide many technical problems too difficult to overcome under local anesthesia. c) the operating room manners of the surgical team are critical for the outcome of the operation and a calm atmosphere is a necessity. d) some patients are too ill to receive general anesthesia and could be deprived the benefits of a needed carotid endarterectomy if not for local anesthesia.

We feel that local anesthesia is a safe and effective operative approach to the management of cerebral ischemia and, at the same time, a most accurate, cost-effective method for neurologically monitoring the patient. Thus we advocate the teaching of the technique to vascular trainees.

References

1. Hertzer NR (1988) Presidential address: Carotid endarterectomy – A crisis in confidence. J Vasc Surg 7: 611–619
2. Garraway M, Connolly DC, Elveback LR, Whinsant JP (1983) The dichotomy of myocardial and cerebral infarction. Lancet 2: 1223–5
3. Rutkow IM, Ernst CB (1986) An analysis of vascular surgical manpower requirements and vascular surgical rates in the United States. J Vasc Surg 3: 74–83
4. Forssell L, Takolander R, Bergqvist D, Bergentz SE, Olivecrona H (1988) Risk Factors in Carotid Artery Surgery: An Evaluation of 414 Operations. Ens J Vasc Surg 2: 9–14
5. Baker WH, Dorner DB, Barnes RW (1977) Carotid endarterectomy: Is an indewelling shunt necessary? Surgery 82: 321–6
6. Hafner CD, Evans WE (1988) Carotid endarterectomy with local anesthesia: Results and advantages. J Vasc Surg 7: 232–9
7. Rich NM, Nobson RW (1975) Carotid endarterectomy under regional anesthesia. Amm Surg 4: 253–9
8. Imparato AM, Ramirez A, Riles T, Mintzer R (1982) Cerebral protection in carotid surgery. Arch Surg 117: 1073–8
9. Connolly JE (1985) Carotid endarterectomy in the awake patient. Amm J Surg 150: 159–63
10. Evans WE, Hayes JP, Waltke EA, Vermillion BD (1985) Optimal cerebral monitoring during carotid under local anesthesia. J Vasc Surg 2: 775–7
11. Liapis CD, Satiani B, Florance CL, Evans WE (1981) Motor speech malfunction following carotid endarterectomy. Surgery 89: 56–9
12. Meec AC, Chidlow A, Lane IF, Greenhalgh RM, McCollum CN (1988) Platelet kinetics following Carotid Endarterectomy. The Effect of Aspirin and Patch Angioplasty. Eur J Vasc Surg 2: 99–104

Author's address:
Prof. Christos Liapis, MD, PhD
Athens University Medical School
131, Vas. Sofias
11523 Athens, Greece

Intraoperative assessment of cerebral ischemia: somatosensory evoked potentials, transcranial Doppler and oxymetry

S. Horsch, K. Ktenidis, Ch. Konstantis, C. Bartels

Department of General and Vascular Surgery, Krankenhaus Porz am Rhein, Academic Teaching
Hospital of the University of Cologne, Germany

Present-day discussions amongst specialists show that carotid surgery has to stand up to constantly increasing demands. Apart from strict guidelines for surgical indications as well as involved surgical technique, the necessity of perioperative monitoring is increasingly stressed.

The monitoring during carotid reconstructions is particularly demanded. The significance of this monitoring consists of the evaluation of the clamping effect, determination of the neccessity of using a shunt, evaluation of the effectiveness of the shunt, timely recognition of intraoperative complications and the insurance of operative quality.

Intraoperative measurement of stump-pressure in the internal carotid artery and electroencephalography were monitoring devices that have been used since the end of the 1960s. Because of their lack of reliability and the immense technical and personal display, vascular surgeons started to look for new methods (1, 3) and somatosensory evoked potentials (SEP) and transcranial Doppler ultrasound (TCD) were introduced. In 1994, we introduced transcranial cerebral oxymetry as another monitoring method in carotid surgery.

Whereas SEP and EEG allow intraoperative monitoring of the brain function (2, 5), stump-pressure control and TCD deliver information about intracerebral hemodynamics (4). Transcranial oxymetry measures the regional cerebral oxygen saturation in the cerebral blood during clamping period.

The aims of the monitoring procedures were:
▶ the quantitative determination of the risk of cerebral ischemia during the clamping period and the necessity of an intraluminal shunt
▶ the registration of intraoperative complications as embolisation or dysfunctional shunt.

Material and methods

From January 1990 until February 1992, we monitored brain function during carotid endarterectomy of 1295 patients during 1411 operations in our clinic using SEP and/or TCD (571 female, 724 male; average age 64.3 years). SEP were derived from the ipsilateral cortex after stimulation of the contralateral median nerve at the wrist. Electrodes were placed in the middle of the forehead behind the ear and at a distance of 4 x 2 cm away (parietooccipital) from this point. According to the literature and our experience the loss of SEP's or the N20/P25 amplitude reduction of more than 50 % was determined as abnormal. TCD was performed transtemporally as described by AASLID. The flow-velocity was measured in the main branch of the middle cerebral artery (MCA). Based on own experiments the reduction of mean flow-velocity of more than 70 % was determined as critical point for the TCD method.

From February 1994 until September 1994, we included 136 patients in another study, who underwent 148 carotid endarterectomies. The mean age was 67 years (range 50–81). There were 82 men and 54 women. Within the contex of this prospective comparative study, we monitored transcranial cerebral oxymetry (TCO) and somatosensory evoked potentials (SEP) during carotid surgery. The aim of the study was to determine the use of transcranial cerebral oxymetry as an additional monitoring device in carotid surgery. We used the SEP as reference value. Using the two mentioned methods, we monitored 148 carotid reconstructive procedures in the above period. The transcranially determined regional O_2 saturation was determined in the temporofrontal brain tissue up to depth of 50 mm using near-infrared-spectroscopy (INVOS 3100, Somanetics, Troy, MI). The reduction of regional O_2 saturation of more than 10 % is considered as abnormal, based on animal and a few human studies. The regional cerebral oxymetry is a measure of the percentage saturation in the brain's vascular bed. It is a sensitive parameter for determining the relation between oxygen supply and oxygen consumption in the brain. Due to the effect of predominantly venous blood in the cerebral vascular bed, the oxygen saturation measured primarily represents the cerebral venous circulation.

Results

The data analysis of the total number of cases (n = 1411) found the following results: The performance or the evaluation of SEP (TCD) monitoring failed in 7.8 % (66.8 %) of all cases.

Because abnormal SEP/TCD monitoring the intraluminal shunt was inserted in 19.2 % of cases. In the postoperative period (before discharge) we registered new neurological events in 4.3 % (TIA: 1.4 %, RIND: 1.8 %, stroke: 1.1 %). The mortality rate was 1.5 %. The cause of death was the stroke in 0.9 %, the cardiac and pulmonary failure in 0.6 %. The sensitivity and specificity of SEP/TCD monitoring is 100 % and 98.9 %. We found positive and negative predictive values of 100 % and 99.8 %.

The statistical analysis of the "OXYMETRY-study" (n = 136) found a sensitivity of 97.6 % and specificity of 66.6 %. Twelve cases showed abnormal cerebral oxygen saturation and somatosensory evoked potentials. In three cases we registered abnormal SEP, but normal oxymetry. In these cases we inserted an intraluminal shunt. The rate of shunting was 9.3 % (n = 15). Despite shunting, three of these patients suffered an intraoperative neurological deficit (one stroke, two TIA's). Two other patients developed neurological deficits (TIA, RIND) postoperatively. We see the sequential cerebral oxygen changes during the important phases of operation. After clamping of the carotid artery the oxygen saturation is usually reduced by about 5–8 %. At the end of the operation we often see a short-term increase of the rSO2 because cerebral reperfusion. The abnormal oxymetry is demonstrated on this figure. After the clamping the oxygen saturation is always reduced more than 10 %. After the placement of an intraluminal shunt we see a clear increase of saturation. In all abnormal cases we did not notice the complete normalization of oxymetry, but at the end of clamping, we registered a complete normalization.

Discussion

The risk of cerebral ischemia during the clamping period is always present during carotid surgery. In agreement with most vascular surgeons, we consider intraoperative monitoring important and necessary. The existing methods with an established high reliability are SEP and EEG. Alternatively, surgery under local or regional anaesthesia is possible.

Our results showed that the observation of the somatosensory evoked potentials is the superior procedure (sensitivity and specificity over 95 %) as monitoring method in carotid surgery.

Intraoperative TCD monitoring delivers useful information about the effect of clamping on intracranial hemodynamics. TCD alone is not useful in detecting intraoperative complications such as embolization. These lesions are located within the very peripheral branches of the middle cerebral artery, however specialists do not agree on the critical point of flow reduction during the clamping period.

The cerebral regional O_2 saturation seems to be an additional useful monitor. This method shows acceptable reliability (sensitivity: 97.7 %, specificity: 66.6 %). Further advantages were: the simplicity of the method, non-invasive and continuous monitoring, and no additional personnel requirement.

References

1. Branston NM, Symon L, Crockard HA et al. (1974) Relationship between the cortical evoked potential and local cortical blood flow following acute middle cerebral artery occlusion in the baboon. Exp Neurol 45: 195
2. Amantini A, Baretelli M, de Scisciolo G et al. (1992) Monitoring of somatosensory evoked potentials during carotid surgery. Neurology 239: 241
3. Dawson GD (1947) Cerebral responses to electrical stimulation of peripheral nerve in man. J Neurol Neurosurg Psychiatry 10: 134
4. Dinkel M, Schweiger H, Goerlitz P (1992) SEP monitoring during carotid surgery versus carotid stump pressure. J Neurosurg Anesth 4: 167
5. Horsch S, Ktenidis K, Ricke S et al. (1995) Intraoperative quality assessment during supra-aortic surgery. Langenbecks Arch Chir Suppl Kongressbd 1084–1086

Author's address:
Prof. Svante Horsch, MD, PhD
Krankenhaus Porz am Rhein
Chirurgische Klinik
Lehrkrankenhaus der Univ. zu Köln
Urbacher Weg 19
51149 Köln, Germany

Current therapeutical concept of carotid occlusive disease

U. Weiher

Department of Thoracic and Vascular Surgery, 1. Hospital IKA, Athens, Greece

The incidence of stroke in the USA and Europe is about 200/100000 population per annum and increases in patients > 75 years old to 1440/100000, while the yearly incidence of death caused by stroke is 5–10 % of all deaths (1–3). About 60 % of survivors remain disabled (4). The costs for all the patients with cerebrovascular diseases in the United States is 15 billion dollars/year and are still increasing. Nearly 40–50 % of all the strokes are caused from occlusive disease of carotis bifurcation (4).

All patients with carotis-stenosis have to be treated with the best medical therapy, which includes: stop smoking, optimal therapy of diabetes, reduction of blood pressure, reduction of weight and hyperlipidemia, and last but not least, antiplatelet – or anticoagulant therapy. In several trials there was no difference in therapeutic efficacy between Acetyl-sylicyclacid (ASA) and anticoagulants (AC) (5, 6), while the therapy with ASA or Ticlopidin is easier and cheaper. Ticlopidin is probably more effective than ASA, but has more adverse effects (leucopenia) (7). Common practice is to consider AC if antiplatelet therapy fails and there is no indication for operation (7). Heparin is given intravenously in patients waiting for the operation with filiform stenosis or TIA's in evolution.

Our question is, which patients have to be treated operatively, mainly by classical Carotid endarterectomy (CEA) and Eversion-CEA- but in singular cases possibly also with endovascular procedures in case of fibromuscular dysplasia or very peripher stenosis, where CEA is not indicated, even if it is very disputed (8).

CEA has been proposed as a stroke-preventing treatment, the frequency of its use increased in the 1970s and 1980s, and peaked in 1985 with 107000 CEA in the USA; thereafter the frequency declined so that in 1990 only 60000 where performed, because of the uncertainty of its benefit. This was subsequently evaluated in large randomized clinical multicenter-trials, comparing the surgical risk and benefit with those of not operating.

The North American Symptomatic Carotid Endarterectomy Trial (NASCET) showed that the risk of ipsilateral stroke in the medical treated patients was 26 % within 2 years vs. 9 % in the surgical treated. The perioperative major stroke and death rate was 2 % and the mortality 1 %. The efficacy of operation in stenoses > 70 % was proved in February 1991 and the trial was stopped for this group, but it is still on going for patients with stenosis < 70 %. No data in this trial have yet confirmed benefit of CEA in stenosis < 70 % (2).

The European Carotid Surgery Trial (ECST) had a perioperative (30 days) morbidity and mortality 3.7 %, but in the following years the rate of disabling or fatal stroke was 2.8 % annually vs. 16.8 % in the medical group. In this trial, too, the efficacy of CEA was early proved in severe (> 70 %) stenosis. In mild (0–29 %) stenosis there is no benefit of operation. The NASCET and ECST continue for moderate (30–69 %) stenosis, first results are expected in 1996–97.

The patients with ulcerated plaque have an indication for CEA also with stenosis < 70 %, because the deep ulcer nearly doubles the risk of stroke (1, 12, 13).

In cases of prior stroke with minimal deficit the incidence of recurrent stroke is quite high 9–16 %/year and can be reduced with the CEA to 2 %/year. It is advised to perform the operation 4–6 weeks after the neurological event and not later than 3 months (12, 13).

The indication in asymptomatic patients is much more controversial and uncertain. The CASANOVA study (Carotid Artery Stenosis Asymptomatic Narrowing: Operation Versus Aspirin) could not prove a benefit of CEA in stenosis 50–90 %. Patients with higher stenosis were excluded from the trial. Although one of the participants of the trial advises to operate 80 % stenosis, considering that one of the centers which participated had a too-high morbidity and mortality and changed the results of the entire trial (15).

The Veteran Affairs Cooperative Trial (VACT) find benefit in operated patients in all grades of stenosis > 50 %, even if it was proved only in consideration of the stroke incidence but not the mortality incidence (16). The ACAS (Asymptomatic Carotid Atherosclerosis Study) which randomized until February 1993, 1500 patients, has not yet sufficient data to report a result. Currently in progress in Europe is the Asymptomatic Carotid Surgery Trial (ACST). In conclusion, most authors agree to operate 80 % stenosis, especially if there exists an ulcerated plaque or a contralateral occlusion, which may quadruple the risk of stroke (13). It seems to be useful to perform a stress EKG or stress scan with thallium before CEA because of the high incidence of Coronary Artery Disease (CAD) reaching 35–40 % in patients with ICA-stenosis (18).

In cases of global ischemia CEA seems to have a benefit if the stenosis is bilateral 75 % or occlusion of one ICA is present (3). The chronic occlusion will not be operated ipsilaterally, but the contralateral stenosis will be corrected. The acute occlusion especially as a result of CEA, has a certain indication for immediately operation.

The management of patients scheduled for Coronary Artery Bypass (CAB) with stenosis of A. carotis is not standarized. Schlosser, for example, will not perform CEA in asymptomatic stenosis; in symptomatic patients he does so 7–10 days before CAB, and in case of unstable angina pectoris, he operates simultaneously (17). Gilling-Smith advises to also operate asymptomatic stenosis if there is present occlusion of one ICA or high bilateral stenosis or infarcts in CT of brain (18). They agree there is no evidence that CEA will reduce perioperative stroke.

Recurrent stenosis is treated like primary ones if it is a clearly atherosclerotic stenosis. The early recurrent stenosis caused by myointimal hyperplasia can be treated conservatively, because a remains mostly asymptomatic until 70–80 % stenosis.

In conclusion, there is a clear indication for CEA in symptomatic stenosis > 70 % independent of the morphology of the plaque. Symptomatic stenosis < 70 % with ulcerated plaque and asymptomatic stenosis 80 % are also to be operated. However the guidelines of the American Heart Association should be followed that the perioperative morbidity and mortality must not to exceed 3 % in asymptomatic patients, 5 % in TIA, 7 % in prior stroke and 10 % in recurrent stenosis, while the mortality has to be less than 2 %.

References

1. Toole JF (1993) Asymptomatic Carotid Atherosclerosis Study, in Greenhalgh-Hollier RM: Surgery for Stroke, London, pp 352ff
2. Naslet (1991) Benefit Effect of Carotid Endarterectomy in Symptomatic Patients with high grade stenosis. N Engl J Med 325: 445–453
3. Moore WS et al. (1992) Carotid Endarterectomy: Practic guidelines; Report of the ad hoc committee of the Joint council of the Society for Vascular Surgery and the North American Chapter of the International Society of Cardiovascular Surgery. J Vasc Surg 15: 469–479
4. Rose FC (1993) Epidemiology of Stroke. In: Bernstein EF et al.: Cerebral Revascularisation, London, pp 5ff
5. Sze PC et al. (1988) Antiplatelet agents in the secondary prevention of stroke. Stroke 19: 436–442
6. Jonas S (1988) Anticoagulant treatment in cerebrovascular disease. Stroke 19: 1043–1048

7. Thomas D (1993) Medical Therapy in Patients with carotid Bifurcation Disease. In: Bernstein EF et al.: Cerebral Revascularisation, London, pp 197ff
8. Kachel R (1993) Endovascular Treatment of Carotid and Vertebral Arteries. In: Bernstein EF et al.: Cerebral Revascularisation, London, pp 661ff
9. Carotid Endarterectomy for Asymptomatic Carotid Stenosis (1993) N Engl J Med 328: 276–278
10. ECST Collaborative group (1991) MRC European Carotid Surgical Trial: interim results for symptomatic patients with severe (70–99 %) or with mild (0–2 %) carotid stenosis. Lancet 337: 1236–1243
11. Müller-Wiefel H (1992) Carotis-Chirurgie: Indikation zur Operation – Wann operieren und wann beobachten? Angio 14, Nr. 6: 239–242
12. Money SR, Hollier L (1993) Indication for Carotid Endarterectomy According to Presenting Clinical Symptoms. In: Greenhalgh RM, Hollier LH: Surgery for Stroke, London, pp 97ff
13. Barnett HJ (1993) Status report on the NASCET. J Mal Vasc 18: 202–208
14. CASANOVA study group (1991) Carotid Surgery Versus Medical Therapy in Asymptomatic Carotid Stenosis. Stroke 22: 1229–1235
15. Hamann H (1992) Früh- und Spätergebnisse der Carotischirurgie. Angio 14, Nr. 6: 243–248
16. Veteran Affairs Cooperative study group (1993) Carotid Stenosis. N Engl J Med 328: 221–227
17. Schlosser V (1993) Cerebral artery disease and concomitant coronary heart diseases, simultaneous or staged approach. In: Bernstein EF et al.: Cerebral Revascularisation, London, p 671ff
18. Gilling-Smith GL, Wolfs JH (1993) The Management of Asymptomatic Carotid Disease in Patients who Require Coronary Artery Bypass. In: Greenhalgh RM, Hollier LH: Surgery for Stroke, London, pp 107ff
19. Moore WS (1993) Recurrent carotid stenosis. In: Bernstein EF et al.: Cerebral Revascularisation, London, pp 327ff
20. Coselli JS, Total occlusion of the Internal Carotid Artery: an approach to treatment

Author's address:
Ursula Weiher, MD
Department of Thoracic and Vascular Surgery
1. Hospital IKA
Zaimi Street
15127 Melissia, Athens, Greece

Operative results after carotid endarterectomy

K. Balzer

Department of Vascular Surgery, Evangelical Hospital Muehlheim on the Ruhr, Germany

Introduction

According to the NASCET-study, the Veterans-Administration-study, as well as the European study, the discussion concerning the indication for operative treatment of carotid artery stenosis which lasted over years, may be regarded as completed. The impressive results showed that the operative intervention is of less risk for the patient than the natural history. The multicentre studies have been negatively influenced by some high figures from participating centres. Nevertheless, with a clear percentage < 3 % concerning operative morbidity and mortality the benefit of the vascular surgery can be proved. In discussing this subject, one fact is frequently omitted: the perioperative risk figure is augmented especially by that group of patients who will not be able to gain any profit by the vascular surgical management due to their advanced stage III or IV, which results consequently in a high rate of complications.

Indication for operation

Operative indication should follow careful clinical examinations including the consideration of symptoms. Therefore noninvasive screening tests, particularly Doppler-ultrasound-sonography and Duplex scanning are of decisive importance. By means of Duplex scanning the morphological diagnosis of arteriosclerosis will be made and so the risk of embolisation following soft-plaques can be determined. Apparently calcified hard-plaques are less dangerous in spite of a high degree of stenosis. Angiography may be ommited in cases where the carotid stenosis is unmistakably identified. In the cases of symptomatic carotid stenosis, but usually also in asymptomatic stenosis, a CT-scan for the clarification of unnoticed ischemic insults or the differential diagnosis of a multiinfarct syndrome is indispensable. Transcranial Doppler ultrasound is a proven method for the screening of the collateral perfusion. Age and accompanying diseases are a less important factor for the operative indication.

Operative technique

The surgical approach must follow for good exposure of the arterial region in question. This is best done by an incision made at the anterior margin of the stenocleidomastoid muscle. After sufficient preparation of the vessels and clamping, a short arteriotomy is made to open the common carotid artery and is extended into the internal carotid artery until an undiseased segment of the artery is reached and the stenotic plug can be visualized and dissected in its entirety. The incision has to be extended far enough into the internal carotid artery, so that a possible resulting distal step from an endarterectomy can be tacked with atraumatic suture to prevent a dissection. Disobliteration often leads to distinct elongation of the vessel if cleavage has taken place between the outer layer of the media and the adventitia. This must be corrected in every case. Endarterectomy of the internal carotid artery is continued into the common carotid artery. If the atheromatous plug with an inner core containing intima and media does not taper off at its proximal end, it must be sharply divided, leaving a small ledge behind. Retrograde application of the ring stripper may be unsafe and hazardous and will not remove the thickened intima without leaving a ledge or injuring the artery at its origin. In this case the reconstruction must be carried out under proximal preparation under controlled circumstances.

The dissection of the stenotic layer might already be done under the insertion of an intraluminal shunt. The introduction of the shunt enables the reconstruction of the cerebral circulation. Whether or not a shunt should be added is still debated. The results of the teams working without a shunt are not inferior to those who generally use a shunt. In between is the group of elective shunters who make their decision to use a shunt or not depending on evoked potentials and EEG-monitoring with trend-analyser or transcranial Doppler. We personally only insert a shunt if corresponding changes in the EEG or evoked potentials are seen, or if the transcranial Doppler indicates a critical ischemia or complete occlusion of blood flow in the medial cerebral artery. Great care should be taken not to inflict any injury or embolisation when inserting the shunt. A premature clamping is good protection against peripheral embolisation and better than the disadvantages of long clamping times. All protective measurements formerly undertaken have failed.

The closure of the arteriotomy is usually done with a patch graft. Either an autogenous vein, harvested from the great saphenous vein above the medial malleolus, or a synthetic patch may be used. It also might be done by a direct suture, which leads however to a higher restenosis rate. It is of importance to review the external carotid artery, otherwise an occlusion of this vessel may occur. More dangerous is the case when such a ledge may extend into the internal carotid artery with a postoperative thrombosis.

For some years the new method of eversion endarterectomy has been available. After transection of the internal carotid artery the adventitial layer is turned upside down over the stenosing plug. It is important to consider adversion of a distal intimal flap, which is why angioscopy after surgical procedure is mandatory to control the lumen of the vessel. More-or-less long incisions of the arterial stumps allow a shortening of elongations. It is not necessary to implant synthetic material. After early scepticism the new method has become more and more popular.

Results

Based on a prospective study on 600 patients, we were able to find remarkable advantages for the eversion technique. Nevertheless, the figures turned out to be too small to demonstrate statistical significance, but the review of a retrospective analysis on 5000 patients proved the advantages of this method. Therefore, we do believe the eversion endarterectomy is the method of choice whenever possible as opposed to the conventional operative technique.

Concerning the results we would like to refer to the perspectives of the two operative procedures. Irrespective of the selected procedure, the highest risk exists in stage III and IV. The stages I and II indicate a complication rate of < 2 % in the group of the conventional technique. In the group of eversion endarterectomy, however, we found that none of the patients in these stages died or suffered from a permanent neurological deficit.

Transitory neurological disorders with paralytic symptoms, loss of speech, etc. were found in the group of thrombendarterectomy with a rate of 8 %, in the eversion group with a rate of 3 %. These damages disappeared completely after 1 day and are most likely due to the clamping of the cerebral perfusion. The clamping time in the group of the conventional method is ~ 0.5 h, and in the group of the eversion technique approx. 16 min. A correlation of clamping time and postoperative neurological findings is most likely.

In the group of conventional endarterectomy, 9 % had to be reoperated because of postoperative bleedings. This percentage was considerably lower in the eversion group. EEG-changes could be seen more often for conventionally operated patients with a rate of 12.2 %, as in the group of the eversion with only 4.9 %. A shunt was used in 6.5 % of the conventional cases compared to 2.8 % in the eversion group respectively. Certainly it is more difficult to insert a shunt using the eversion technique.

A postoperative examination with ultrasound-Doppler and Duplex scanning showed a relatively high figure (11.4 % conventional endarterectomy, 9.2 % eversion endarterectomy) of intimal hyperplasia, which was seen during the first 6 months, but not followed later by real recurrent stenoses. The postoperative examination after 6 months showed no essential differences regarding the long-term results of the two different methods. Recurrent stenoses could be proved at 3.8 % of the conventionally operated and 3.9 % of the eversion group. After 1 year < 1 % in both groups suffered from transitory ischemic attacks (TIA). One stroke occurred during 2 years in the eversion endarterectomy group. According to the lifetable analysis, 93 % of the TEA-group and 95 % of the eversion group survived the first year, with 88 % and 90 % respectively in the second year. By omitting the stages III and IV the results improve to 96 % for the first year and 92 % for the second year of the two groups. All deaths were due to cardiac failure with the exception of one deadly stroke. Two patients died due to cancer.

Conclusions

Reasonable results are reported by all experienced centres. Surgery on the carotid artery may be noted of significant advantage compared to the conservative therapy, which is always included in the operative treatment. This can be adequately proven by actual studies. By restricting the complications to the stages I and II, in our experience a percentage of < 2 % is seen concerning the conventional technique. No complications were observed by using eversion endarterectomy in these stages. This underlines not only the advantage of the surgical management in stage II, but also in the asymptomatic stage I. The good results of the eversion endarterectomy indicate the benefit of this surgical technique, which should be used whenever possible.

The perioperative monitoring is of high importance. We prefer evoked potentials or the EEG with trend-analyser. Certainly the success of the surgical management depends on the skill and experience of the surgeon. This allows an extended indication in the future when considerating Duplex scanning and in regarding the type of the atherosclerotic disease. The long-term morbidity and mortality is less in the stages I and II, highlighting the importance of the prophylactic operation in time. Most patients died because of cardiac failure. Stroke is, as seen by this study, a rarely seen postoperative complication. The safety of the patient demands a sufficient diagnostic procedure as well as a consequent indication. Both are as important as good surgical and postoperative management.

Karos in the Greek language means heavy sleep. The old Greeks called the arteries of the neck 'carotid arteries', because they believed that when they were pressed hard the man became sleepy. According to a legend, the Centaur fought against a soldier using the technique of pressing the carotid artery and was thus seen to be winning the fight. From the vascular surgical point of view we should do our best to ensure that the name for this artery does not represent its meaning. In other words, fighting against stroke by safe operative technique and vascular reconstruction in time.

References

1. Aburahma AF, Robinson P, Decanio R (1989) Prospective clinicopathologic study of carotid intraplaque hemorrhage. Am Surg 55: 169–173
2. Balzer K, Carstensen G (1985) Rekonstruktionen an der A. carotis. Ökonomie der Diagnostik und Ergebnisse. Dtsch Med Wochenschr 110: 510–512
3. Brott T, Thalinger K (1984) The practice of carotid endarterectomy in a large metropolitan area. Stroke 15: 950–955
4. Carstensen G, Balzer K (1986) Die asymptomatische Carotisstenose: Wann soll – wann muß man – wann soll man nicht operieren? Langenbecks Arch Cir 369: 97–103
5. Casanova Study Group (1991) Carotid surgery versus medical therapy in asymptomatic carotid stenosis. Stroke 22: 1229–1235
6. Cebul RD, Whisnant JP (1989) Carotid endarterectomy. Ann Intern Med 111: 660–670
7. Chambers BR, Norris JW (1984) The case against surgery for asymptomatic carotid stenosis. Stroke 15: 964–967
8. Diener HC, Dichgans J, Gundalin J, Seboldt H, Huth C, Hoffmeister HE (1984) Asymptomatische Karotisstenose: ist die operative Insultprophylaxe noch gerechtfertigt? Med Klin 84: 128–132
9. Hennerici M, Hülsbömer HB, Hefter H, Lammerts D, Rautenberg W (1987) Natural history of asymptomatic extracranial arterial disease. Brain 110: 777–791
10. Hobson RW, Weiss DG, Fields WS, Goldstone J, Morre WS, Towne JB, Wright CB and the Veterans Affairs Cooperative Study Group (1993) Efficacy of carotid endarterectomy for asymptomatic carotid stenosis. N Engl J Med 328: 221–227
11. Kasprzak PM, Raithel D (1990) Eversionsendarterektomie der Arteria carotis interna (EAA). Angiology 12: 1–8
12. Kasprzak PM, Raithel D (1989) Eversion carotid endarterectomy. Technique and early results. J Cardiovasc Surg 30: 49
13. Marx P (1990) Therapiekonzept bei asymptomatischer Karotisstenose: Operationsindikation aus neurologischer Sicht im Vergleich zum Spontanverlauf. Langenbecks Arch Chir, Supp I, Verh Dtsch Ges Forsch Chir: 537–542
14. North American Symptomatic Carotid Endarterectomy Trial Collaborators: Beneficial effect of carotid endarterectomy in symptomatic patients with high-grade carotid stenosis: J Med 7
15. Norris JW, Zhu CZ, Bornstein NM, Chambers BR (1991) Vascular risks of asymptomatic carotid stenosis: Stroke 22: 1485–1490
16. Towne JB, Weiss DG, Hobson RW (1991) First phase report of cooperative Veterans Administration asymptomatic carotid stenosis study-operative morbidity and mortality. J Vasc Surg 11: 252–258
17. van Dongen RJAM (1984) Angiographische Pathomorphologie der A. carotis aus chirurgischer Sicht. In: Mahler F, Nachbuhr B (eds) Zerebrale Ischaemie. Huber, Bern, pp 125–129
18. Vollmar J (1982) Rekonstruktive Chirurgie der Arterien. Georg Thieme-Verlag, Stuttgart, New York

19. Widder B (1987) Transkranielle Doppler-Sonographie bei zerebrovaskulären Erkrankungen. Springer-Verlag, Berlin Heidelberg New York Tokyo
20. Widder B, Kornhuber HH (1987) Wann ist die Carotisoperation noch indiziert? Dtsch Med Wochenschr 112: 405–407
21. White DN, Curry GR (1977) Colour coded differential Doppler ultrasonic scanning system for the carotid bifurcation. Experta Medica, Amsterdam/Oxford
22. Zhu CZ, Norris JW (1991) A therapeutic window for carotid endarterectomy in patients with asymptomatic carotid stenosis. Can J Surg 34: 437–440

Author's address:
Dr. Klaus Balzer
Chefarzt der Gefäßchirurgischen Klinik am Evangelischen Krankenhaus
Wertgasse 30
45468 Mülheim an der Ruhr, Germany

Carotid endarterectomy without preoperative angiography

E. Bastounis, Chr. Maltezos, P. Balas

First Surgical Department, University of Athens, Greece

Summary

Three-hundred-and-twenty-eight endarterectomies of the carotid artery in 328 patients were carried out from January 1, 1987 to December 1994 in the 1st Surgical Dept, University of Athens Medical School. There were 243 males (82.93 %) and 50 (17.07 %) females. The mean age of the above patients was 67.5 years. One-hundred-and-forty-four endarterectomies were done without preoperative angiography; instead ultrasonography using Duplex or Triplex scanning was used, while in the remaining 184 endarterectomies an angiographic investigation of the carotids was performed. This study was undertaken to compare the postoperative results, the mortality and morbidity in the first 30 days postoperatively as well as their postoperative complications, which showed that the difference between the two groups was not statistically significant. The surgical findings as regards the stenosis rate and texture of the atheromatic plaque together with the corresponding preoperative data are also compared.

The results compiled up to the present date show that the ultrasonographic control of the carotids can establish exactly the indications for endarterectomy of the carotid artery and, many times, the angiographic study is not necessary for the assessment of the occlusive changes of the carotid bifurcations.

Introduction

It has been generally accepted that atherosclerotic lesions of the extracranial segment of the carotids and carotid bifurcation are the main cause of most cerebrovascular episodes.

Until recently, preoperative angiography of the aortic arch and its branches was the examination of choice to demonstrate their atherosclerotic lesions. The angiographic findings combined with the history, the clinical condition and the age of the patient were enough to define the indications for the carotid endarterectomy (5, 16).

However, with the progress of the noninvasive diagnostic methods, especially ultrasonic (Duplux, Triplex) imaging, it is now possible to have an accurate preoperative picture of carotid bifurcations and their atherosclerotic lesions without performing angiography.

In the last decade many authors have compared the two diagnostic methods (angiography-ultrasonographic study) regarding the indications of carotid surgery. Nevertheless, there are a good number of authors who claim that the preoperative control of the carotids with only ultrasonography is an amply accepted and safe method, with high specificity and sensitivity for the demonstration of atherosclerotic plaques of the carotid bifurcation (2–4, 6–14) (Table 1).

Table 1. Early results of carotid endarterectomy performed without preoperative angiography

Authors	No of cases	Stroke	Perioperative TIA	Event
Blackshear et al., 1982	4	0 (0.0%)	0 (0.0%)	0 (0.0%)
Sandmann et al., 1983	91	0 (0.0%)	0 (0.0%)	0 (0.0%)
Gonzalez et al., 1984	5	0 (0.0%)	0 (0.0%)	0 (0.0%)
Crew et al., 1984	65	1 (1.5%)	1 (1.5%)	2 (3.0%)
Thomas et al., 1986	32	0 (0.0%)	0 (0.0%)	0 (0.0%)
Marshall et al., 1988	26	1 (3.8%)	1 (3.8%)	2 (7.6%)
Moore et al., 1988	32	0 (0.0%)	0 (0.0%)	0 (0.0%)
Hill et al., 1990	130	1 (0.7%)	2 (1.4%)	3 (2.1%)
Wagner et al., 1991	255	6 (2.4%)	0 (0.0%)	6 (2.4%)
Total	640	9 (1.4%)	4 (0.6%)	13 (2.0%)

Collaborators 1991; European Carotid Surgery Trialists' Collaborative Group, 1991; Mayberg et al. 1991

The present investigation deals with 130 patients who were subjected to carotid endarterectomy using only Duplex or Triplex, in order to study, preoperatively, the carotid bifurcation and to compare the results of an equal number of patients who had undergone preoperative angiographic control of the carotids during the same period of time.

Materials and methods

During the period from January 1 1987 to December 31 1994, 328 carotid endarterectomies were performed in a total number of 293 patients (35 patients had been subjected to bilateral carotid endarterectomy) in the 1st Surgical Department, University of Athens Medical School.

Two-hundred-and-forty-three (82.93 %) of the patients were males and the remaining 50 (17.07 %) females. The mean age of the patients was 67.5 years.

One-hundred-and-thirty patients (Group A) were subjected to carotid endarterectomy based on the Triplex or Duplex scanning findings only, while the remaining 163 (Group B) had undergone a selective angiography of the aortic arch and its branches in order to study the carotid bifurcations (Table 2).

If the ultrasonic examination had been performed in a period of more than a week before surgery, a repeat examination was done, mainly in severely stenosed carotids, the

Table 2. Carotid endarterectomies (from 1.1.1987 to 31.12.1995)

	Group A*	Group B**
No of operations	144	184
No of patients	130	163
Male	105 (80.76 %)	138 (84.66 %)
Female	25 (19.24 %)	25 (15.84 %)

* Group A: without angiography; ** Group B: with angiography

day before operation, in order to exclude a complete occlusion which might have occurred in the meantime as had happened in several of our cases.

All the patients had a preoperative brain CT scan and clinical neurological evaluation. The ultrasonographic examination of the carotids was performed by the same experienced examiner in all our cases.

In many cases a cardiac examination was performed including echocardiography, myocardial thallium scintigraphy or Holter monitoring. In addition, all patients had a complete coagulation profile workup.

Regarding the risk factors of the patients, 87 % were smokers or had been smokers in the past, 72 % were hypertensive, while 26 % were diabetics.

Of the 130 patients of group A, 40 (30.76 %) were asymptomatic (without a history of TIA or stroke), while the remaining 90 patients (69.24 %) had a history of neurological symptomatology.

Of the asymptomatic patients, 22 (55 %) had a negative CT brain scan for infarct while 18 patients (45 %) presented with a "silent" cerebral infarct; in the patients of group A, 23 (17.69 %) presented with total occlusion of the carotid on one side and stenosis ≥ 50 % on the other.

Of the patients of group B, 52 were asymptomatic (31.9 %) while 111 (68 %) were symptomatic. Of the asymptomatic patients, 28 (53.84 %) were negative for preoperative CT findings of the brain, while 24 (46.16 %) were positive for findings. Twenty-nine patients of group B (17.79 %) presented with total carotid occlusion on the one side and stenosis ≥ 50 % on the other (Tables 3, 4).

Table 3. Symptomatology

Symptomatology	Group A	Group B	Total
Symptomatic	90 (69.23 %)	111 (68.09 %)	201
Asymptomatic	40 (30.76 %)	52 (31.91 %)	92
Complete occlusion on one side, stenosis ≥ 50 % on the other side	23 (17.69 %)	29 (17.79 %)	52

Table 4. Indications according to symptomatology

Symptomatology	Group A		Group B	
	No	%	No	%
Asymptomatic CT scan (−)	22	16.92	28	17.17
CT scan (+)	18	13.84	24	14.72
T.I.A.	60	46.15	79	48.46
Symptomatic with neurologic deficit	25	19.23	28	17.17
Amaurosis fugax	5	3.84	4	2.45
Complete occlusion on one side Stenosis ≥ 50 % on the other side	23	17.69	29	17.79

Thirty-two % of patients of group A and 28 % of patients of group B had a bilateral neck murmur while 72 % of patients of group A and 69 % of patients of group B had a neck murmur on one side only.

All patients were subjected to carotid endarterectomy by the same surgical team. General anesthesia was administered to all patients and a shunt between common and internal carotids was used. A venous patch from the patient's major saphenous vein was placed after endarterectomy in 120 patients of group A (92.3 %) and 158 (96.93 %) patients of group B; in the remaining patients a synthetic patch was used.

Results

Of the 144 carotid endarterectomy procedures of group A patients there was an "agreement" between the diagnostic-ultrasonographic and surgical findings as to the stenosis rate of the carotid bifurcation and the texture of the atherosclerotic plaque by 92 %. Only in nine cases was there "disagreement" between the preoperative-ultrasonographic data and surgical findings. Approximately the same rate of agreement was found between the preoperative-diagnostic data and surgical findings in patients of group B (91.4 %) as regards the rate of stenosis, while in this second group regarding the texture of the atherosclerotic plaque there was no significant information.

The total postoperative morbidity for patient groups A and B was 4.26 % for the 30 first days while the total mortality rate was 1.52 % (Table 5).

Analytically, the morbidity rate for patients of group A was 3.47 % while the corresponding rate of patients of group B was 4.89 % ($p > 10$ %).

It was 2.08 % regarding the mortality rate for group A patients while for group B patients the rate was 1.08 % ($p > 10$ %) (Table 6).

The causes of death in group A patients was: One patient sustained extensive, severe cerebrovascular episode with damage to the brain stem, another patient had an extensive myocardial infarct while the third patient sustained rupture of the venous patch. In group B patients the two deaths were due to severe cerebrovascular episodes.

The general and local complications for groups A and B patients are classified in Tables 7 and 8. Four weeks postoperatively one of the patients of group A (0.76 %) had a thrombosis of the carotid bifurcation which subsided asymptomatically.

Table 5. Immediate surgical results (within 30 days)

	Morbidity		Mortality	
	Group A	Group B	Group A	Group B
Asymptomatic	–	2	1	2
Symptomatic	3	5	2	–
Complete occlusion on one side, Stenosis ≥ 50 % on the other side	2	2	–	–
Total per group	5	9	3	2
Total		4.26 %		1.52 %

Table 6. Immediate surgical results (within 30 days)

	Group A No of operations: 144		Group B No of operations: 184	
	No	%	No	%
Morbidity	5	3.47	9	4.89
Mortality	3	2.08	2	1.08

Cause of death:

Group A		Group B	
Stroke	1	Stroke	2
Myocardial infarction	1		
Rupture of venous patch	1		

Table 7. General complications

Complications	Group A		Group B	
	No	%	No	%
Hypertension	4	2.77	4	2.17
Hypotension	8	5.55	12	6.52
T.I.A.	6	4.16	8	4.34
Myocardial Ischemia	1	0.69	1	0.54
Neurological deficit	2	1.38	5	2.71

Table 8. Local complications

Complications	Group A		Group B	
	No	%	No	%
False aneurysm	–	–	1	0.54
Venous patch rupture	1	0.69	–	–
Horners' syndrome	1	0.69	1	0.54
Hypoglossal nerv lesion	1	0.69	1	0.54
Laryngeal nerv lesion	1	0.69	–	–
Facial nerv lesion	3	2.08	2	1.08

Discussion

Selective angiography of the aortic arch and the carotids was considered by almost all vascular surgeons and angiologists as the "point of reference" of imaging techniques for the diagnosis of atherosclerotic changes of the carotids and for decision-making of carotid endarterectomy. However, since 1982, when Blackskear et al. (1) carried out their first carotid endarterectomy without preoperative angiography, a new chapter has come up in the preoperative diagnostic evaluation of the occlusive changes of the carotid bifurcations.

A good number of carotid endarterectomies have been performed in the recent years in various centers in the USA with amply successful and encouraging results, without the use of preoperative angiography (2–15).

Perioperative morbidity and mortality in the above series are mostly comparable and smaller than those of corresponding series of endarterectomies with preoperative angiography (4). This fact establishes our experience up to the present data (2, 3).

Despite the above, there was and there still exists scepticism among vascular surgeons as to the safety which is offered by only preoperative ultrasonographic control in assessing the atherosclerotic lesions on the carotid bifurcations.

How safe is the preoperative ultrasonographic control of the carotids and which are the advantages and disadvantages of the method over elective angiography? It is, first of all, a less expensive, noninvasive and easily prepared diagnostic method with almost equal and/or more precise results than that of angiography, mainly when it concerns stenoses greater than 60 – 80 %. In Goodson's (17) series of 78 carotid endarterectomies, the sensitivity of ultrasonography was very impressive (99 %) over 91 % of arteriography (p = 0.06). Ultrasonography gives better information regarding the texture of the atherosclerotic plaque (hard, soft, etc.), the existence of ulcer or thrombus or the existence of hemorrhage within the plaque, factors which are in close relationship with the indications for carotid endarterectomy (6–8, 11, 17).

It is worthwhile mentioning that elective angiography gives us ample information concerning the occlusive atherosclerotic changes of the carotid bifurcations (extension and degree of stenosis starting from the common to the internal carotid), for any possible existing anatomical anomalies of the internal carotid artery, the existence of intracranial aneurysms or other lesions (5, 16).

In order to recognize the lesions of the intracranial branches of the carotids there exist possibilities of controlling these lesions by ultrasonography using special "windows" in the skull. However, this method is not considered very precise and safe as compared to the angiographic control of the intracranial branches. It has now been accepted that better angiographic imaging is obtained by selective intraarterial carotid imaging where we can examine any possible lesion existing from the origin of the carotids arising from the aortic arch as far as the carotid bifurcations and even beyond them, as well as up to the intracranial branches.

And now the question arises of how safe is this method?

Intraarterial imaging is an invasive method requiring hospitalization and with certain risks. Hankey et al. (9) in a recent investigation of over 8300 subtraction angiographies reported an incidence of neurological deficit 24 h after surgery at a rate of 4 % with a remaining neurological deficit of 1 % and a mortality rate of 0.1 %. On the other hand, the possibility of existing systematic or local complications at a rate of 0.5 % – 9.4 % and 0.6 % – 20.8 % respectively, dictate the need for contemplation whether the ultrasonographic preoperative control of the carotids constitutes a much better alternative. On of the disadvantages of the ultrasonographic method is that its results are in closer relationship with the examiner than that of angiography, and that imaging of the lesions is done for the part of the carotid which is situated a little before or after the bifurcation.

The careful clinical examination and the discovery of murmurs at the supraclavicular, intraclavicular or neck area, may dictate the need of additional angiographic checking.

The view has been entertained, that these patients who presented with atherosclerotic lesions in sites of the internal carotid, over the bifurcation (tandem lesions), constituted a contra-indication for endarterectomy and revascularization. These lesions may, however, be shown only by angiography and not by ultrasonography, in which case may escape observation.

The answer to the above theory was given by Moore et al. in 1988 (13), in studies which showed that "tandem lesions" of the internal carotid, beyond the bifurcation, do not constitute a contra-indication for revascularization with carotid endarterectomy, a fact which shows that angiography would absolutely not have been indispensable for patient selection.

As regards the meager possibility of ultrasonographic control of the intracranial branches and the existence of possible angiodysplasias or other lesions, CT or MRI (when required) gives an answer to many questions.

As it results from other reports and protocols and the authors' experience, the need for CT brain scanning preoperatively, in patients with carotid stenoses, to check the existence of "silent" or asymptomatic infarcts is imperative, as opposed to the opinion of Martin et al. (12).

According to the opinion of Wagner et al. (14), more than 70 % of patients who present with carotid stenosis might sustain surgery based only on ultrasonographic data.

In conclusion, the experience of our unit up to the present date, that assessment of the carotid bifurcation with a proper clinical examination is a reliable ultrasonographic control in a high-tech center, by the same experienced examiner, assisted by CT brain scanning or MRI (when required), pose the indications for carotid endarterectomy with ample preciseness and safety.

References

1. Blackshear WM, Connar RG (1982) Carotid endarterectomy without arteriography. J Cardiovasc Surg 23: 477–482
2. Balas P, Bastounis E, Pangratis N, Xeromeritis N, Masouridou E (1994) Carotid endarterectomy without cerebral arteriography. Intern Angiol 13: 18
3. Balas P (1992) Are the ultrasonic imaging technics (duplex or triplex) alone sufficient for decision-making in carotid endarterectomy? Pros and Cons Intern Angiology 2: 91–93
4. Crew JR, Dean M, Johnson JM et al. (1984) Carotid surgery without angiography. Am J Surg 148: 217–220
5. Dowson DL, Zierler RE, Kohler TR (1991) Role of arteriography in the preoperative evaluation of carotid artery disease. Am J Surg 161: 619–624
6. Flanigan DP, Schuter JJ, Vogel M et al. (1985) The role of carotid duplex scanning in surgical decision making. J Vasc Surg 215–225
7. Giender JW, Lampavello PJ, Rites TS et al. (1989) Is duplex scanning sufficient evaluation before carotid endarterectomy? J Vasc Surg 9: 193–201
8. Gerther JP, Cambia RP, Kistler JP et al. (1990) Carotid surgery without arteriography: Non-invasive selection of patients. Ann Vasc Surg 4: 253–256
9. Hankey GJ, Warlow CP, Sellar RJ (1990) Cerebral angiographic risk in mild cerebrovascular disease. Stroke 21: 209–222
10. Hill JC, Carbonneau K, Baliga PK et al. (1990) Safe extracranial vascular evaluation and surgery without preoperative arteriography. Ann Vasc Surg 4: 34–37
11. Leahy AL, McCollum PT, Feeley MC (1988) Duplex ultrasonography and selection of patients for carotid endarterectomy: Plaque morphology or luminal narrowing? J Vasc Surg 8: 558–562
12. Martin JD, Valentine RJ, Myers SI et al. (1991) Is routine CT scanning necessary in the preoperative evaluation of patients undergoing carotid endarterectomy? J Vasc Surg 14: 267–270
13. Moore WS, Ziomek S, Quinones-Baldrich WJ et al. (1988) Can clinical evaluation and noninvasive testing substitute for arteriography in the evaluation of carotid artery disease? Ann Surg 208: 91–94
14. Wagner WH, Treiman RL, Cossman DV et al. (1990) The diminishing role of diagnostic arteriography in carotid artery disease: Duplex scanning as definite preoperative study. 15th Annual Meeting of the Peripheral Vascular Surgery Society, June 2, L. Angeles-Calif

15. Pedrini L, Paragona O, Disano E et al. (1991) Morbidity and mortality following carotid surgery. J Cardiovasc Surg 32: 720–725
16. Ricotta JJ, Holen J, Schenk E et al. (1984) Is routine angiography necessary prior to carotid endarterectomy? J Vasc Surg 1: 96–102
17. Goodson SF, Flanigan DP, Bishara RA, Schuler JF, Kikta MS, Mayer JP (1987) Can carotid duplex scanning supplant arteriography in patients with focal carotid territory symptoms? J Vasc Surgery 5: 551–557

Author's address:
Prof. Elias Bastounis, MD, PhD
"Laiko" General Hospital
17, Ag. Thoma St.
11527 Athens, Greece

Carotid endarterectomy without patch and shunt

V. Andrikopoulos

Department of Vascular Surgery, "KAT" General Hospital, Athens, Greece

Cardiovascular diseases, according to the data from the Ministry of Health in 1992, are the leading cause of death in Greece with a mortality rate of 50 %. Half of those deaths (25 %) are caused by stroke. With a decreasing frequency, malignant neoplasms account for 21 % of deaths, traffic accidents for 5 %, etc.

The annual current incidence of stroke is approximately 20000 (two strokes per thousand of the population), 15000 of which are due to lesions of the extracranial vessels (75 %) and 7500 lead to death.

Although there is agreement that carotid endarterectomy is the most effective prophylactic method in the management of patients with arteriosclerotic lesions of the carotid arteries, there is still much controversy about the best means of protecting the brain from embolism and ischemia during carotid clamping.

Analysis and comparison of results after endarterectomy in an attempt to define the best method of brain protection is difficult due to the following factors:

▶ Great variation of preoperative clinical symptoms ranging from a simple dizziness to complete hemiparesis which makes grouping of patients impossible.
▶ Diversity of carotid stenosis morphology.
▶ Variety of means for brain protection from ischemia.
▶ Adequacy of intracranial collateral circulation.
▶ Small number and variety of neurological complications.

Several studies have dealt with the critical questions whether measurements of brain tolerance are necessary and whether cerebral blood supply during the period of temporary carotid occlusion should be increased.

The controversy about these subjects strongly suggests that there is no method which nullifies complications. Thus, the use of a shunt either blindly or after some brain tolerance measurements is an important part of the surgery and assures adequate cerebral blood circulation.

However, some vascular surgeons do not favor its routine use and many questions still require to be answered. Is shunting necessary? Is it safer to perform carotid endarterectomy with the use of a shunt? Are postoperative complications due to embolic phenomena rather than ischemic strokes during clamping time? Are the methods which estimate brain tolerance and subsequently dictate shunt usage safe and reliable?

In the present study patients were selected on the basis of unilateral carotid lesions alone and were grouped according to preoperative symptoms in an attempt to evaluate the efficacy of endarterectomy without shunt and patch.

The surgical approach was endarterectomy under general anesthesia without vessel manipulations such as insertion of shunt, stump pressure measurement, use of patch, based on the concept that optimal results can be obtained by a simple method which does not cause embolism *per se.*

The localized lesion and the simplicity of the surgical procedure minimize the risk of embolization due to causes other than the method itself.

Patients and methods

From January 1987 through December 1994, 144 patients with carotid stenosis were treated in the Vascular Surgery Department of KAT Hospital. Ninety-eight patients (70 males and 28 females) with age ranging from 52 to 74 years (mean age 67 years) who suffered from unilateral atherosclerotic carotid stenosis underwent endarterectomy. Age itself was not a contra-indication to operation.

The remaining 46 patients with concomitant lesions from the intracranial vessels detected by angiography, lesions from the vertebrobasilar system evaluated clinically and angiographically and patients with contralateral hemodynamically symptomatic carotid stenosis were excluded from the study.

All 98 patients had no neurological deficit prior to operation and were classified in three stages based on clinical symptoms:

Stage I: 18 asymptomatic patients with stenosis of more than 70 %.

Stage II: 72 patients with TIA only.

Stage III: 8 patients who have had a stroke with good recovery (TRINS). Of those, 2 presented bruit and 6 TIA.

The preoperative diagnostic workup included Duplex sonography, CT brain examination and four vessel angiography with visualization of the intracranial vessel system.

Based on the sonographic findings the patients were subdivided into the following categories:

A) 18 patients with carotid stenosis of 50–80 %
B) 50 patients with carotid stenosis of more than 80 %
C) 30 patients with atherosclerotic ulcerations

Operative management

All operations were performed under normocarbic general anaesthesia, with continuous monitoring of ECG and blood pressure. Induced hypertension during the clamping time was controlled with Ringer's solution.

The surgical technique was atraumatic and carotid dissection was handled with utmost gentleness. One cc of heparin intravenously (5000 Units) was administered 3 min before carotid clamping. The adequacy of collateral circulation was evaluated by visual assessment of the back flow from the internal carotid.

Flushing of all debris and air from the arteriotomy site was performed routinely. The ECA was opened first, followed by the ICA. Neither shunt nor patch was used and closure of the arteriotomy was performed with a 6/0 or 7/0 running monofilament suture.

Clamping time ranged from 8 to 29 min with an average of 17.04 min. Hypertensive attacks were managed with glyceryl trinitrate (Nitro-lingual inf.) or Nitroprusside infusion. Heparin was not reversed.

In brief, shunt, patch, EEG or stump pressure measurement were not used.

Postoperative care

All patients were mobilized the first postoperative day and received a salicylate tablet (325 mg/day). Discharge from the hospital took place between the 7th and 10th postoperative day.

Results

A. Operative morbidity

Complications were grouped as follows:

I. Surgical complications: such as infection, hematoma and nerve paresis (Vagus, hypoglossal, and marginal branch of facialis).

II. Internal complications: myocardiac infarction, stenocardia etc.

III. Neurologic deficits (permanent or temporary)

Acute: due to intraoperative embolism. They occurred immediately after the patient awakened from general anesthesia.

Delayed: which developed within a period of 10 days as a result of thrombosis of the endarterectomy, intracerebral hemorrhage, edema, hyperperfusion syndrome, hypertension or hypotension. In these cases patients awakened intact and experienced a neurologic deficit either immediately after or later during the postoperative period.

B. Mortality

Patients who died within 10 days after operation (hospitalization period).

No mortality or internal complications were noticed in our series. Two cases of wound hematomas did not cause problems.

The overall neurologic morbidity of 5 % consisted of 2 (2 %) permanent and 3 (3 %) temporary deficits.

Acute neurological deficits: There were two acute neurological deficits, one of which was permanent and one temporary, clearing up within 24 h (both from clinical stage II with TIA).

Delayed neurological deficits: There were three delayed deficits, two of which were temporary, clearing up within 24 and 48 h respectively, and one was permanent.

The three delayed deficits developed in patients who belonged in clinical stage III.

All neurological complications, exept one, developed in patients with ulcerated plaque detected by Duplex (category C, in our study).

There seemed to be no correlation between clamping time and neurological complications.

Discussion

Carotid endarterectomy has become the established therapy for patients with atherosclerotic lesions.

In the present study the selection of patients with unilateral carotid lesions alone, the classification into clinical groups and the use of a simple method enabled us to decide whether or not the use of a shunt is necessary or in other words whether ischemia or embolism is the main cause of the acute neurological deficits.

The reasons that encouraged us to perform endarterectomy under normocarbic general anaesthesia without means of brain protection are the following:

a) Local anaesthesia causes lesser degree of comfort for the patient and the surgeon. Postoperative strokes cannot be ruled out even in patients who tolerate a test occlusion of 3 min and finally the increased oxygen demands in patients under local anaesthesia may increase the hazard of cerebral hypoxia (1–4). The increased sympatho-adrenal response and metabolic requirements make the use of local anaesthesia in patients with cardiac disease undesirable.

b) Hypothermia has proved to cause serious cardiac arrythmias (5).

c) Hypercarbia inceases total cerebral blood flow (CBF), but autoregulation at a low pressure state is absent and the cerebral vessels are unresponsive to an increased pCO_2. Thus an intracerebral steal phenomenon to the advantage of the contralateral hemisphere occurs (2).

d) Electroencephalographic monitoring includes a substantial number of both false positive and false negative results and does not correlate with the clinical outcome (6). The EEG under local anaesthesia can be normal during a profound neurological deficit while EEG changes indicating ischemia can be found in patients with normal neurologic response (1).

e) Patch angioplasty according to our experience and to the results of other studies causes a significant enlargement of the vessel lumen resulting in increased turbulence and lack of a laminar flow (7).

f) The use of a shunt into the arteriosclerotic vessel has among others some inherent disadvantages (embolic events, intimal flaps, tears, obscurity of the proximal and distal limits of the plaque, peri shunt thrombosis, malfunction). The occurrence of neurological complications does not significantly differ in patients who underwent endarterectomy with or without shunt. Thompson and Talkington (8) and Thompson et al. (9) who routinely employed a shunt in 1666 endarterectomies report a mortality rate of 2.4 % and a stroke rate of 1.4 % while Whitney et al. (10), in a series of 1917 patients operated without a shunt, report a mortality rate of 1.9 % and a stroke rate of 3.3 %.

Whether the selective use of a shunt with carotid stump pressure measurement is the best solution remains to be determined and the views on the critical level of stump pressure differ (11). According to some authors stump pressures of 50 to 55 mmHg or higher reflect adequate cerebral collateral circulation, while others have set a pressure of 25 mmHg as a critical threshold (8). This discrepancy may be partially due to the differences in brain O_2 demands during local and general anaesthesia and to the use of induced systemic hypertension. On the other hand, complications can occur even with a shunt and a stump pressure of more than 50 mmHg (8). Finally, in using stump pressure one must also consider the factor duration of carotic clamping. A stump pressure which may be safe for a short period of occlusion may not be safe for an unexpected long period of occlusion (12).

The transcranial Doppler technique is very sensitive to the small changes in middle cerebral artery blood flow, but low velocity changes as well as the adequacy of the collaterals cannot be assessed.

Finally, we are not experienced with other sophisticated techniques such as monitoring of somatosensory potentials, infra-red cerebral oximetry (13), etc.

The trial of normocarbic general anaesthesia undertaken in all our operations is known to increase the tolerance of brain to cerebral ischemia due to decreased metabolic demands for oxygen. Furthermore, general anesthesia is well accepted by both the patient and the surgeon. Induced systemic hypertension which directly influences stump pressure was raised from 20 to 40 mmHg above the preoperative levels during the clamping period.

In our series, mortality rate was zero while postoperative complications included two acute and three delayed neurological deficits. The three delayed deficits could not be attributed to cerebral anoxia that results from cross-clamping the carotid artery, because the patients awakened intact. Of the remaining two acute deficits, one was a permanent stroke (clamping time: 23 min) and the other was a temporary deficit (clamping time: 19 min) clearing within 24 h. These could have been avoided by the use of a shunt under the condition that the risk of a stroke from the shunt itself is nullified.

Although the number of patients in our series is small and statistical analysis of the results is not possible, the following conclusions can be drawn:

The small percentage of permanent neurological deficits (2 %) and the absence of deaths in our series, suggest that endarterectomy without a shunt, at least in cases with no concomitant hemodynamically significant lesions, is a safe method.

All neurological complications, exept one, developed in patients with ulcerated plaques detected by sonography (Duplex).

Clamping time does not seem to correlate with the clinical outcome.

Endarterectomy without a shunt is a safe method in cases with no hemodynamically concomitant significant lesions and the neurological complications are probably due to embolic phenomena rather than temporary ischemia during operation.

References

1. Bergeson P, Benichou H, Dupont M et al. (1989) Carotid surgery under cervical block anesthesia: A simple method of heart and brain protection in high risk patients. Int Angiology 8: 70–80
2. Akl BF, Blakeley WR, Lewis CE, Edwards WS (1975) Carotid endarterectomy: Is a shunt necessary? Am J Surg 130: 760–765
3. Buford AW, Keats AS, Cooley DA (1977) Increased tolerance to cerebral ischemia produced by general anesthesia during temporary carotid occlusion. Surgery 54: 216–226
4. Takdander R, Bergqvist D, Hulthen V, Johansson A, Katzman P (1990) Carotid artery surgery. Local versus general anesthesia as related to sympathetic activity and cardiovascular effects. Eur J Vasc Surg 4: 265–270
5. Baker WH, Darner DB, Barnes RW (1977) Carotid endarterectomy: Is an indwelling shunt necessary? Surgery 82: 321–326
6. Forssell C, Takolander R, Bergqvist D (1990) Pressure measurements as predictors for preoperative neurologic deficits in carotid surgery. Eur J Vasc Surg 4: 153–158
7. Hirschi M, Bernt RA, Hirschi MM (1989) Carotid endarterectomy (CE) of the internal carotid artery (ICA) with and without patch angioplasty: Comparison of hemodynamical and morphological parameters. 8: 10–15
8. Thompson JE, Talkington CM (1976) Carotid endarterectomy. Ann Surg 184: 1–15
9. Thompson JE, Austin DJ, Don Patman R (1970) Carotid endarterectomy for cerebrovascular insufficiency. Long-term results in 592 patients followed up to thirteen years. Ann Surg 172: 7663–7679
10. Whitney DG, Kahn EM, Estes JW, Jones CE (1980) Carotid artery surgery without a temporary indwelling shunt. Arch Surg 115: 1393–1399
11. Kwaan JHM, Peterson GJ, Connolly JE (1980) Stump pressure: An unreliable guide for shunting during carotid endarterectomy. Ann Surg 115: 1083–1085
12. Naylor AR, Wildsmith JAW, McDure J, Jenkins A (1991) Transcranial Doppler monitoring during carotid endarterectomy. Br J Surg 78: 1264–1268
13. Panetta TF, Legatt AD, Veith FJ (1993) Somatosensory evoked potential monitoring during carotid surgery. In: Surgery for Stroke. Greenhalgh RM, Hollier LH (ed.) WB Saunders, pp 273–285

Author's address:
Vasilis Andrikopoulos, MD
Department of Vascular Surgery
"Kat" General Hospital of Athens
2, Nikis St.,
14561 Kifisia-Athens, Greece

Choice of graft material in carotid surgery: vein versus PTFE

D. Raithel

Department of Vascular Surgery, Nuremberg Hospital, Nuremberg, FRG

Carotid endarterectomy is – despite current controversy – at present one of the most frequent arterial operations performed by vascular surgeons. Some authors prefer primary closure, following carotid endarterectomy (CEA), others prefer patch angioplasty by vein patch or Dacron/PTFE to increase the lumen size of the artery (1–6). Others have chosen a new technique such as eversion endarterectomy or graft interposition (7–11).

The rate of restenosis reported in the literature ranges from 1.2 % to 23.9 %, depending on postoperative invasive or non-invasive surveillance (2, 9, 12–14). Most of these restenoses documented by non-invasive diagnostic techniques were asymptomatic, and only 1.2 to 3.6 % of the cases had to be operated on, due to an asymptomatic restenosis of more than 80 % or symptomatic restenoses.

Our experience in carotid "redo"-surgery has shown excellent results with graft interposition (vein, Dacron or PTFE), so that we have extended our indication even to primary procedures (10).

Indication for graft interposition

We see three main indications for graft interposition: preoperative, intraoperative, and perioperative.

A) Preoperative (elective):

In patients with recurrent carotid artery stenoses an endarterectomy with or without overpatching is not always possible, and therefore we recommend graft interposition by vein or prosthetic material. In aneurysms of the common carotid artery or ICA and in patients with tumors we recommend graft interposition, too.

In patients with significant kinkings of the ICA and with tortuosity we also primarily use graft interposition with vein or PTFE.

In patients with infections after carotid endarterectomy (CEA) we see the indication for autologous tissue and interpose vein segments in carotid position.

B) Intraoperative:

Graft interposition is also indicated intraoperatively in patients with technical problems during endarterectomy. In the earlier series we mostly tried to implant saphenous vein segments. Now we interpose 6 mm PTFE prostheses in nearly all the cases, with the exception of infections.

C) Perioperative (urgent):

Urgent indication for graft interposition is mostly seen perioperatively in patients with postoperative neurological deficit or stroke due to partially or totally thrombosed endarterectomized carotid segments. Furthermore, we see clear indication for patients with postoperative bleedings, in whom reconstructions with suture repair is not possible, and who need graft interposition.

In patients with carotid trauma or with ruptured carotid aneurysms as well as in patients with carotid dissection of the CCA or ICA, graft interposition is indicated.

Material and Methods

Between August 1984 and March 1993, we performed 7824 carotid end-arterectomies at the Vascular Department of the Nuremberg Medical Center. Graft interpositions were used in 154 (2 %) operations: 108 PTFE grafts, 9 Dacron, and 37 vein grafts. For this study we only compared the PTFE- to the vein graft group.

There were 66 men and 76 women with a mean age of 66.9 years in the PTFE group, and 65.6 years in the vein group.

Risk factors include tobacco abuse in 66.9 %, diabetes in 32.4 %, hypertension in 62.1 %, and hypercholesterinemia in 41.4 %. 48.3 % of the patients had coronary heart disease.

Preoperatively, we mostly saw the indication for graft interposition in patients with restenoses; in 43 cases we interposed PTFE grafts, and in three cases vein segments.

Eight patients showed late infections; two of them had infected patch aneurysms, and all these cases were reconstructed by saphenous vein segment interpositions.

Quite frequently, we saw the indication for graft interposition in patients in whom we had technical problems during endarterectomy of the carotid artery (39 patients).

In the perioperative period 20 patients (0.3 % of the CEA and EEA) had to be urgently reoperated due to neurological deficits after carotid endarterectomy. The reasons for these deficits were partially or completely thrombosed endarterectomized segments of the ICA or CCA.

In two patients we had to perform a vein graft interposition after postoperative bleeding; in these patients we were not sure if the bleeding had been caused by an infection, and therefore a vein segment had to be interposed.

The mean clamping time in the PTFE group was 39.8 min., and in the vein group it was 46.6 min.

In all reconstructions with PTFE we used a 6 mm Gore-PTFE graft. In the vein group the mean diameter was 4.3 mm. We performed distal oblique end-to-end anastomosis between the graft and the normal ICA. Therefore the portion of the ICA that was diseased or previously endarterectomized was resected. The proximal anastomosis between the graft and the common carotid artery was done end-to-side at the CCA opposite the external carotid artery (Fig. 1). Pre- and postoperatively all patients received platelet inhibitors (100 mg / per day).

Results

There were four deaths in the total group (2.8 %): two due to permanent neurological deficits, one due to bleeding with operative revision, and one due to myocardial infarctions.

Comparing the three groups we had one death (1.2 %) in group A (preoperative / elective indication), three deaths in group C (perioprative / urgent indication), but no death in group B (intraoperative indication).

In the total group we had two transient (1.4 %) and five permanent (3.5 %) neurological deficits. Analyzing the different groups, we had two transient (2.3 %) and one permanent (1.2 %) deficits in group A. No neurological deficit was seen in group B, but four permanent neurological deficits (20 %) in group C.

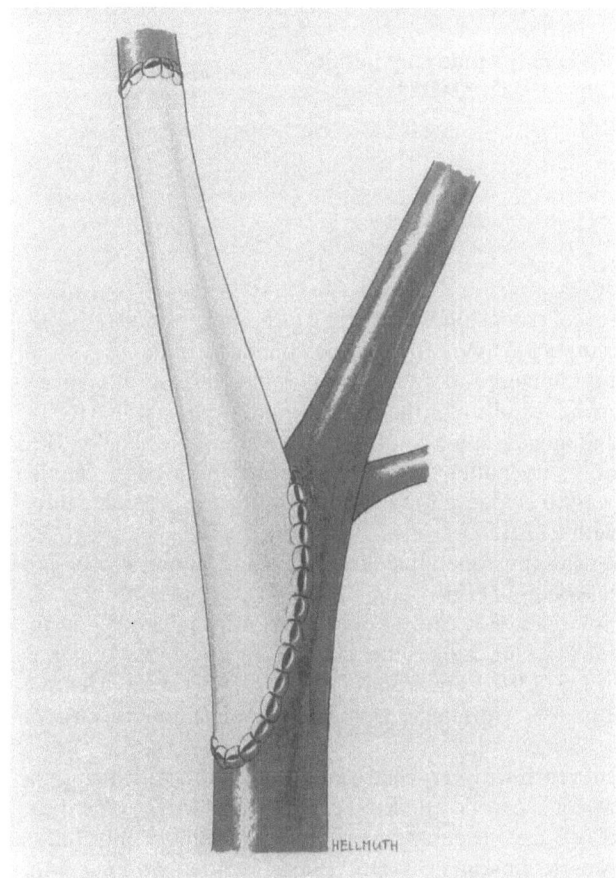

Fig. 1. PTFE or vein graft
interposition in carotid surgery

One vein graft, but no PTFE graft occluded in the perioperative period.

All but three patients operated on with graft interposition were followed-up (mean duration 28.2 months; range 3 to 103 months). During the follow-up period, five patients died, 8 to 40 months after operation. Two of these patients died as a result of complications from stroke, one ipsilateral and one contralateral stroke. The remaining three patients died from causes unrelated to carotid disease (two due to cardiac events, one due to cancer). The follow-up was done by questionnaire, physical examination, and Duplex-scan in all surviving patients. Digital angiography was performed whenever significant recurrent stenoses or contralateral stenoses were suspected.

The late results were excellent: Most of the patients were asymptomatic. Only two new transient ischemic attacks and two strokes had developed in the vein group, and one stroke in the PTFE group.

Graft patency: Only one graft in the vein graft group reoccluded asymptomatically, but none in the PTFE group.

The actual patency rate is 100 % in the PTFE group and 94.6 % in the vein group in a mean follow-up of 28.2 months. We saw two mild restenoses (below 50 %) in the PTFE group and two in the vein graft group. In three patients of the vein graft group a hemo-dynamically significant restenosis (over 50 %) developed, but none in the PTFE group.

Furthermore, two anastomotic aneurysms were seen in the vein graft group. We saw no late infections in either group.

The overall survival rate was 91 % in the follow-up period.

Discussion

In 1988, Mogan et al. presented excellent results with 6 mm PTFE interpositions between the CCA and the ICA in carotid surgery (8). As Mogan joined our department in 1991, we have adopted his experience and implanted more and more PTFE instead of vein segments in carotid position. Our former results plus the current follow-up results have especially convinced us of the fact that angiographic control has shown mild restenoses (less than 50 %) in two patients only; no patient showed a hemodynamically effective restenosis. Furthermore, there was no evidence for anostomotic aneurysms or late infections in our patient population with PTFE.

We did not have any problems such as postoperative suture bleedings either, as occasionally observed when PTFE patches are used (15).

During the 103-month study interval, 7824 carotid operations were performed at the Vascular Department at the Medical Center, Nuremberg. PTFE or saphenous vein graft interpositions were performed in 145 (1.9 %) operations (PTFE in 1.4 %, vein in 0.5 %). Sise et al. interposed PTFE grafts in 6 %, Cormier et al. in 5 % of their carotid reconstructions (11, 16).

Due to our good results in recent years, we interposed 6 mm PTFE grafts with increasing frequency especially in cases in which a carotid endarterectomy was not safe at the distal intimal point. Since many years, we have used an angioscope for quality control after carotid endarterectomy by eversion technique (17). Due to this angioscopic control the rate of interpositions is higher than in earlier years. By the images obtained in a consecutive series of 196 patients, we found intimal flaps or dissections, which had to be revised, in 3 % (17).

Nowadays these problems are treated by graft interposition, and we use PTFE grafts, because they are easily available, and clamping time is much shorter than when using a vein segment.

The rate of postoperative thrombosis in our series with PTFE was 0 %, and we disagree with Cormier et al. who had 3 % acute postoperative thromboses after PTFE interposition (16). Only two of our patients with vein segment interpositions had a rethrombosis of the graft (one in the perioperative period and one in the follow-up period).

In the follow-up of their series, Sise et al. found an occlusion of the PTFE graft in one patient only (4 %); hemodynamically significant restenosis developed only in two patients (8 %), and two patients (8 %) had a mild restenosis (11). Analyzing their series, they could show that a second restenosis developed in three of nine patients who underwent PTFE interposition graft placement for carotid restenosis. Therefore, their conclusion is that PTFE interposition graft placement for carotid restenosis appears to be a high risk for second restenosis (11). In our series, we could not duplicate these results: We had no restenoses after PTFE interposition in carotid redo surgery (43 reconstructions with PTFE in patients with carotid restenosis).

PTFE may be a reliable conduit for the repair of carotid artery lesions, in cases where routine endarterectomies are not safe or not feasible. These favorable results are due to the fact that these grafts are very short, and the higher flow rates at the carotid bifurcation may be the key factor that these PTFE grafts have a high patency rate (11).

In spite of the excellent results achieved by PTFE grafts they are not statistically different from the vein graft results. In our series with 37 saphenous vein segments with a mean diameter of 4.3 mm of these grafts we had one neurological death with patent vein graft and one ipsilateral stroke, in one of the two patients with a vein graft thrombosis.

The problem with vein interpositions is probably the diamenter of the vein segment. A very narrow diameter is likely to cause rethrombosis, especially when vein segments are used for the correction of recurrent stenosis. Sise et al. reported about three patients with recurrent stenoses in whom they had placed vein interpositions; all of them had early complete reocclusions (11). They also found a few other studies from the literature, and in these studies there were significant rates of recurrent stenosis or total occlusion with saphenous vein segment interpositions (11).

Therefore, we also recommend PTFE interpositions in carotid redo surgery. The interpositions are also a useful alternative to an endarterectomy for unusual lesions such as aneurysms, long segment stenoses with exulceration, and subcranial kinkings with tortuosity. Furthermore, we are convinced that PTFE interposition is mainly indicated in patients who develop thrombosis of the endarterectomized carotid segment in the postoperative period.

We further believe that PTFE grafting offers an advantage in restoring the vessel in a fashion that prevents thromboembolic complications in certain patients in whom arterial closure or endarterectomy is difficult or not safe enough without interposition.

The low restenosis rate of 1.9 % (two patients with a restenosis below 50 %) in the PTFE group justify the use of PTFE in carotid position.

Analyzing our different groups, we had no mortality and no neurological deficit in group B (technical problems during endarterectomy). These results further justify the use of PTFE interpositions, especially in those cases where we do not plan to do it, but we are forced to do it for technical reasons during primary endarterectomy. And there is no need to search for a saphenous vein segment except in patients with an infection.

The PTFE graft is easily available, well adaptive, and has optimal long-term results with no graft occlusion in our series of 108 PTFE grafts so far.

References

1. Clagett GP, Patterson CP, Fisher DF et al. (1989) Vein patch versus primary closure for carotid endarterectomy: A randomized prospective study in a selected group of patients. J Vasc Surg 9: 213–223
2. Eikelboom BC (1993) Carotid Endarterectomy: Patch versus Primary Closure. In Bernstein EF et al. (ed.) Cerebral Revascularisation. London, Los Angeles: Med-Orion Publishing, pp 309–315
3. Lord RSA, Baratha Raj T, Stary DL et al. (1989) Comparison of saphenous vein patch, polytetrafluorethylene patch, and direct arteriotomy closure after carotid endarterectomy. Part I. Perioperative Results. J Vasc Surg 9: 521–529
4. O'Hara PJ, Hertzer NR, Krajewski LP et al. (1992) Saphenous vein patch rupture after carotid endarterectomy. J Vasc Surg 15: 504–509
5. Ouriel K, Green RM (1987) Clinical and technical factors influencing recurrent carotid stenosis and occlusion after endarterectomy. J Vasc Surg 5: 702–706
6. Vanmaele R, Van Schil P, De Measneer M (1990) Closure of the internal carotid after endarterectomy: The advantages of patch angioplasty without its disadvantages. Ann Vasc Surg 4: 81–84
7. Cormier JM, Cormier F, Laurian C et al. (1987) Polytetrafluorethylene bypass for revascularization of the atherosclerotic internal carotid artery: late results. Ann Vasc Surg 1: 564–571
8. Mogán I, Dzsinich Cs, Entz L et al. (1988) Die Interna Interposition als Alternative einer TEA in der Karotis Chirurgie. Angio Archiv 16: 161–162

9. Raithel D (1992) Optimal Technique for Carotid "Redo" Surgery. In Veith FJ ed. Current Critical Problems in Vascular Surgery. vol. 4. St. Louis: Quality Medical Publishing, pp 438–443
10. Raithel D (1993) Current Surgical Techniques of Carotid Endarterectomy. In Bernstein EF et al. (ed.) Cerebral Revascularisation. London, Los Angeles: Med-Orion Publishing, pp 301–307
11. Sise MJ, Ivy ME, Malanche R et al. (1992) Polytetrafluorethylene interpositions grafts for carotid reconstruction. J Vasc Surg 16: 601–608
12. Baker JD (1987) Recurrent Stenosis of the Carotid Artery: Incidence, Diagnosis, Prognosis, and Management. In Moore WS (ed.) Surgery for Cerebrovascular Disease. New York, London: Churchill Livingstone Publishing, pp 703–713
13. Moore WS (1993) Recurrent Carotid Stenosis. In Bernstein EF et al. (ed.) Cerebral Revascularisation. London, Los Angeles: Med-Orion Publishing, pp 327–332
14. Nitzberg RS, Mackay WC, Prendiville E et al. (1991) Long-term follow-up of patients operated on for recuzrrent carotid stenosis. J Vasc Surg 13: 121–127
15. Mc Cready RA, Siderys H, Pittman JN et al. (1992) Delayed postoperative bleeding from polytetrafluorethylene carotid artery patches. J Vasc Surg 15: 661–663
16. Cormier JM, Cormier F, Marzelle J et al. (1993) Polytetrafluorethylene interposition grafts for carotid reconstruction. J Vasc Surg 17: 809
17. Raithel D, Kasprzak P (1992) Angioscopy after Carotid Endarterectomy. Ann Chir et Gyn 81: 192–195

Author's address:
Prof. Dr. med. D. Raithel
Klinik für Gefäßchirurgie
Stadt Nürnberg
KNS/I-3
90340 Nürnberg, Germany

Technique of eversion carotid endarterectomy

D. Kiskinis, N. Saratzis, A. Megalopoulos, V. Dalainas

Department of Vascular Surgery, Achepa Hospital, University of Thessaloniki, Greece

Carotid endarterectomy is well established as a stroke-preventing treatment. Open end-arterectomy performed through a longitudinal arteriotomy is the most common technique for carotid bifurcation endarterectomy. A modification of eversion endarterectomy, however, originally described by Harrison for other arteries (1), can be safely employed for internal carotid endarterectomy. This method does not require longitudinal arteriotomy of the internal carotid artery (ICA) and offers smooth luminal surface throughout the entire length of the vessel.

Eversion endarterectomy has been proposed by Raithel and Kasprzak (2) as a good alternative to open (classical) endarterectomy. However, it has been suggested that this technique is associated with lower restenosis rate and is an optimal method for the correction of an elongated ICA in combination with stenosis (3).

The technique of eversion carotid endarterectomy and our experience is described below.

Technique

Under general anesthesia the patient is placed on the operating table in supine position with the head hyperextended and turned away from the operative side. The skin incision is made parallel to the anterior border of the sternocleidomastoid muscle. Exposure and clamping of the common carotid artery (CCA), external carotid artery (ECA) and ICA are made in the usual way. Systemic heparinization is used. A right-angled bulldog clamp should control the ICA well beyond the distal end of the atheromatous plaque.

The CCA is entered with a scalpel while with an angulated Pott's scissor the arteriotomy is extended in a distal direction toward the fork of the carotid bifurcation.

The incision should be made precisely parallel to the axis of the ECA. A common scissor is then used for complete transection of the ICA. Transection permits complete mobilization of the artery and additional traction downward offers additional length of exposure.

Endarterectomy is started at the stump of the ICA and the plane is developed between the outer most layers of the media and the adventitia.

The atheroma is circumferentially separated and detached while the outer layer of the vessel is everted. Fine atraumatic vascular forceps are required for these manipulations. The eversion is progressively continued distally and the atheroma is detached like a cast. Gentle traction results in complete removal of the atheromatous core providing a thin fading and tapering endpoint. As the atheroma is removed the luminal surface and the transition between endarterectomised and nonendarterectomised segment of the ICA is assessed carefully. Copious quantities of heparinized saline are used to flood the field in order to remove intimal or medial debris. Flaps or loose "residuals" are gently removed only by circumferential traction since cephalad traction can cause inadvertent intimal dissection of the ICA endpoint.

At the next step endarterectomy of the ECA and CCA is attempted. Circumferential mobilization of the plaque is achieved by utilizing the closed jaws of a dissector. After proximal division of the plaque the endarterectomy is carried out into the ECA orifice as far distal as possible.

The arterial wall of the ICA is drawn proximally and the reimplantation of the artery to its normal position is started. The anastomosis begins at the bifurcation fork using a simple running 6–0 synthetic monofilament suture. The posterior wall is reconstructed first with tiny bites.

Prior to completion of the anterior wall of the anastomosis, all clamps are removed sequentially to allow back bleeding and to wash out any thrombogenic debris.

At this stage of the procedure dilators of appropriate size, up to 4.5 mm in diameter, may be used to dilate the extracranial segment of the ICA. Angioscopy may be also used to verify the anatomic result. Angioscopy yields an excellent visualization of the whole endarterectomized luminal surface and the end point of the ICA. After completion of the anastomosis, the blood flow is restored first to the ECA and then to the ICA.

Discussion

During the last 2 years, 88 eversion carotid endarterectomies were performed in our department without perioperative mortality. The permanent stroke rate was zero. No postoperative carotid thrombosis occurred in any patient. During the same period we also performed 226 open endarterectomies with a mortality rate of 1.3 % and a stroke rate of 2.6 %. These results support the concept that eversion endarterectomy is a safe procedure. This method can be employed for ICA endarterectomy even in centers without extensive experience in carotid surgery like ours.

Kasprzak and Raithel in a randomized prospective study compared eversion to conventional (open) endarterectomy (3). A group of 99 patients underwent eversion and another group of 105 patients underwent open carotid endarterectomy. There was no difference in the perioperative mortality and morbidity rate. However, during a mean follow-up of 30 months, an asymptomatic hemodynamically significant carotid stenosis was found in one patient from the eversion group and in eight patients from the open group. They concluded that the occurrence of restenosis was significantly lower after eversion carotid endarterectomy.

The advantage of this technique over the open endarterectomy is that longitudinal arteriotomy of the ICA is avoided and subsequently the suture line does not interfere with the lumen of the vessel. Furthermore, the use of patch in patients with small arteries, such as women and children, is not necessary.

This method is appropriate for the correction of coiling, kinking or tortuosity of the ICA in the presence of arteriosclerotic lesions. After completion of the endarterectomy a segment of appropriate length of the ICA is resected and the vessel is reimplanted.

Among disadvantages of the method is the limitation for an internal shunt placement when it is required. During the step of the eversion endarterectomy of the ICA only a CCA to ECA shunt can be easily used for cerebral protection.

In some complex cases, when the transition end point of the ICA is not smooth and/or the plaque is extented distally, replacement of the ICA by a graft may be necessary. In such cases interposition of synthetic or saphenous vein grafts may be used. There are reports of interposition of polytetrafluoroethylen (PTFE) grafts in carotid circulation with excellent results (4). In one of our patients replacement of the ICA by a 6 mm PTFE graft was required because of unsatisfactory endarterectomy result. The graft remain patent 8 months postoperatively.

In conclusion, eversion endarterectomy is a feasible and safe alternative technique for the management of extracranial carotid arteriosclerosis. The major advantages of this technique are optimum correction of an elongated ICA, lower restenosis rate and avoidance of use of patch material for arteriotomy closure.

References

1. Harrison JH, Jordan WD, Perez AR (1967) Eversion thromboendarterectomy. Surgery 61: 26
2. Kasprzak PM, Raithel D (1989) Eversion carotid endarterectomy. Abstract J Cardiovasc Surg 30: 49
3. Kasprzak PM, Raithel D (1992) Carotid eversion endarterectomy vs conventional endarterectomy. Abstract of the VI annual meeting of ESVS. Athens-Greece, Sept, pp 60
4. Cormier JM, Cormier F, Laurian C et al. (1987) PTFE bypass for revascularization of the atherosclerotic internal carotid artery. Ann Vasc Surg 1: 564–571

Author's address:
Prof. Dimitrios Kiskinis, MD, PhD
53, Hermou St.,
54623 Thessaloniki, Greece

Surgery of the elongated carotid artery – indication, technique, results

K. Ktenidis, L. Claeys, K. Heye, Ch. Konstantis, S. Horsch

Department of General and Vascular Surgery, Krankenhaus Porz am Rhein, Academic Teaching Hospital of the University of Cologne, Germany

Introduction

The surgical treatment of elongations, kinks and coils of the carotid artery is still a major point of debate. Vascular surgeons do not agree on indications for intervention. A further discussed point is the choice of surgical technique (6, 7).

Historical review

The first description of carotid artery was given by Morghani in 1761. The link between carotid kinking and cerebrovascular insufficiency was only noticed by Riser in 1951 (5). He performed a surgical stretching and fixation of the bent arterial segment to the underside of the sternocleidomastoid muscle. However, the patient developed a thrombosis of the anastomotic segment which led to a stroke with fatal consequences. In 1959, Quattlebaum et al. described the first successful reconstruction of a carotid kink (3).

Diagnostics

Apart from a detailed history-taking, the diagnosis requires concise clinical investigations (inspection, palpation and reproduction of patient-described symptoms by putting the cervical spine through its full range of movement. Non-invasive techniques (Doppler ultrasound, B-Scan, color Doppler) are of major use in the diagnosis. Definitive diagnosis however results from arteriography which should include standard pictures with the head in ventral position as well as pictures in variable functional head positions. A cerebral computertomography scan (CCT) is obligatory. Transcranial Doppler ultrasound (TCD) adds an important diagnostic aspect to judging the intracerebral hemodynamics pre- and intra-operatively. The somatosensory evoked potentials (SEP) are suitable for the monitoring of cerebral function (neuromonitoring) during reconstruction, especially during the clamping periods.

Indication for treatment

The indication for surgical intervention is without doubt the most disputed point in the treatment of carotid elongations.

Most authors favor the "Metz classification" (Fig. 1) for determining mode of treatment (6, 7). This scheme uses a purely morphological grading, irrespective of the clinical stage or reduction of arterial lumen in the segment of maximal bend (= kink stenosis). This classification considers the angulation of the elongated carotid artery. The Grade I-elongations show according to Metz grading, an angulation between 90 and 60 degrees. The angulation between 30 and 60 degrees defines the grade II-kinkings. Coilings and < 30 degrees-angulations are considered under the grade III-group.

Vollmar used the classification according to Herrschaft (Fig. 2). This grading distinguishes between C- and S-figured carotid kinkings, coilings and elongations with kink stenosis without other differentiation (2, 8).

In our opinion the limiting morphological criterium to decide to operate does not lie in the degree of kinking or vascular elongation in the angiography, but in the amount of stenosis (kink stenosis) demonstrable at the point of maximum vessel curvature. In this way a purely spiral elongation in the carotid artery may for example demonstrate an angulation of less than 30 degrees (Metz III) in two-dimensional angiography without the existence of a significant reduction of arterial lumen (kink stenosis). Furthermore hemodynamic kink stenosis within coilings can be visualized (specifically of the elipsoid type). For this reason we considered the length of obstructed artery within the kink or coil in addition to clinical symptoms in our proposed indications for surgical intervention. We have used the following morphological classification depending on the degree of the curva-

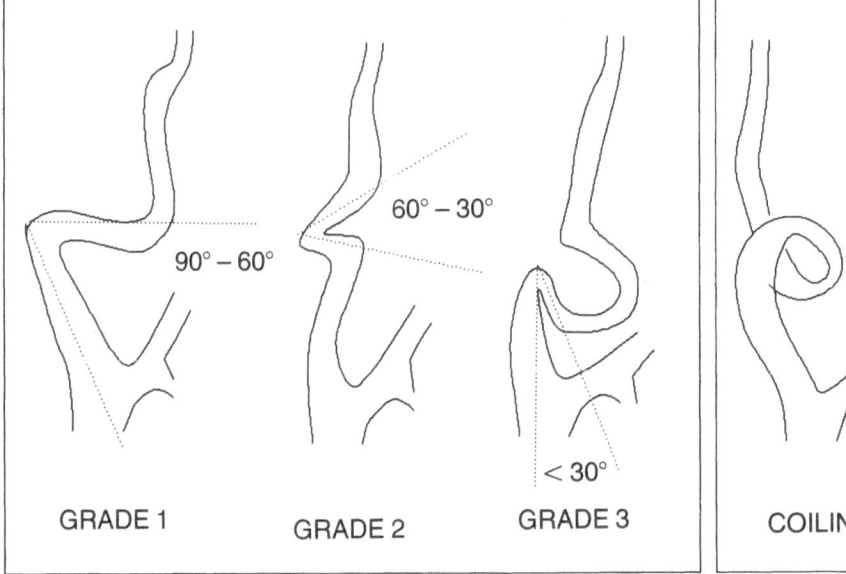

Fig. 1. Classification of carotid angulations according to Metz (1)

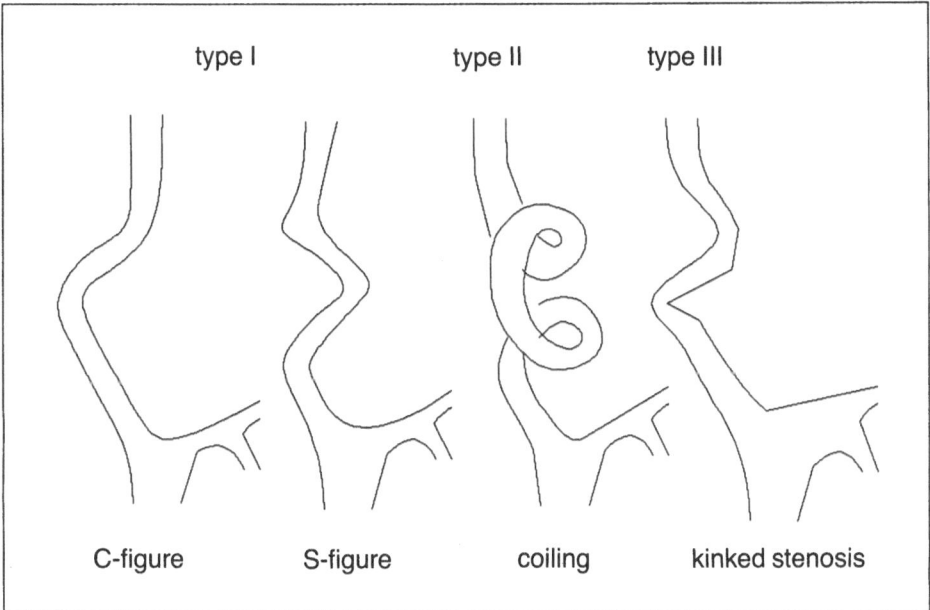

type I   type II   type III

C-figure   S-figure   coiling   kinked stenosis

Fig. 2. Classification of carotid kinking and coiling according to Herrschaft (2, 8)

ture stenosis in the elongated carotid artery, but irrespective of the amount of angulation (Fig. 3). Grade I includes all elongations without angulation stenosis independent of extent or type of elongation; Grade II is composed of elongations with hemodynamic stenostic effects demonstrable under functional head movement.

Low-grade kink-stenosis (less than 60 %) within the elongated vessel form part of grade III. Grade IV incorporates a kink-stenosis of 60–80 %. Those of more than 80 % fall into the fifth category (Fig. 3). The last three grades are angiographically confirmed kink-stenosis, the head being in neutral position with a possible increase in severity of the stenosis by head movements.

An indication for the choice of reconstruction to be used is given by local vessel conditions. Shortening of the elongated artery followed by reinsertion is suitable for S- and C-shaped elongations of different severity. If degenerative vessel wall or small caliber vessels are seen after lengthwise arteriotomy, an expanding patchplasty (vein or PTFE) is indicated. In the case of coilings or spiral elongations resection of the involved segment followed by interposition of a prosthesis (vein or PTFE) is the method of choice. Due to a high risk of causing an iatrogenic dissection of the intima by forceful straightening of kinks or coil, this is advised against (2).

The former method of treatment by altering the elongation and fixing it for example to the sternocleidomastoid muscle is no longer advocated these days and is merely of historical interest (2). The use of an intraluminal shunt is only seldom necessary. Thanks to modern monitoring devices (SEP, TCD). Measuring of residual pressure in internal carotid artery as suggested by some authors has been proven as unreliable.

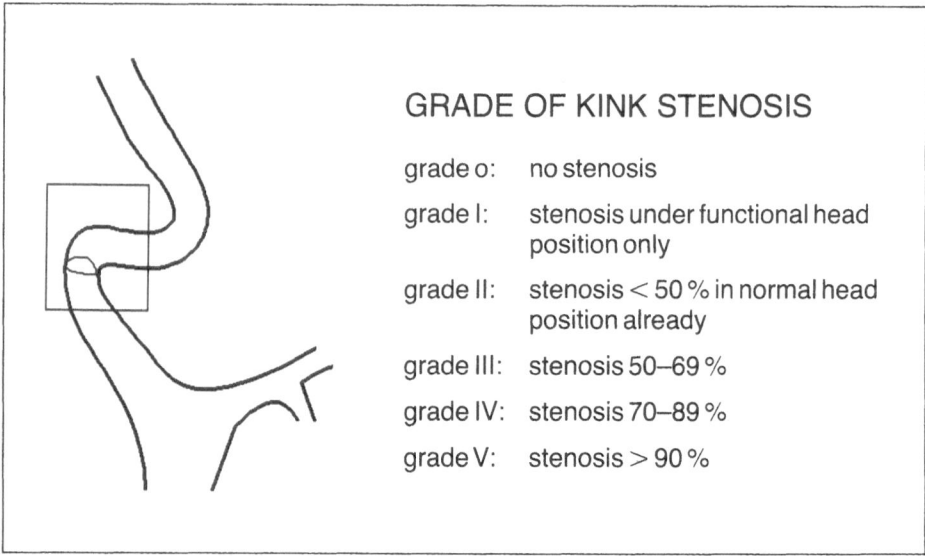

GRADE OF KINK STENOSIS

grade o: no stenosis

grade I: stenosis under functional head
            position only

grade II: stenosis < 50 % in normal head
            position already

grade III: stenosis 50–69 %

grade IV: stenosis 70–89 %

grade V: stenosis > 90 %

Fig. 3. Classification of carotid elongations depending on the degree of the curvature stenosis

Results

In a time span from January 1986 to October 1992, we picked up 49 well-demonstrable elongations in the internal carotid artery region in 42 patients. None of these patients had any obliterating atherosclerosis with this elongation. The mean age was 44 years and the male to female ratio was 1.5:1.

Only 25 of these cases were operated upon and in most of these, resection was followed by reinsertion of the internal carotid artery. In roughly 30 % of cases an additional widening patch angioplasty was performed. In the presence of a coiling (n = 5) this was always resected and a prosthesis (vein or artery) interposed.

Apart from two patients (8 %) with a high-grade but asymptomatic kink stenosis, the indication for surgery was made due to the presence of symptoms (TIA, status after stroke, silent cerebral infraction visible on CT scan). The remaining 24 patients were not treated surgically. The angiographic representation of the elongations not operated on (n = 24) showed elongations of Metz I and II in 91.8 % (n = 22) of cases. Two patients (8.2 %) had a Metz grade III kinking. 38 % of cases (n = 9) of the patients not surgically treated showed no kink stenosis of the elongation by our criteria. Roughly half of the patients showed hemodynamic change in the kink when moving the head into various positions, but without any clinical symptoms. Only three patients had a stenosis more than 50 % with a slight increase in the functional position.

Of the 25 patients operated on 72 % (n = 18) had kinkings of Metz grade III (including of five coiling). 28 % (n = 7) were grade III elongations and 80 % (n = 20) had a kink stenosis within the coil or kink of more than 70 %. In 12 % (n = 3) a symptomatic kink stenosis could only be evoked in functional head position.

The data analysis of the surgically treated patients (n = 25) resulted in the following findings: 72 % of patients (n = 18) had a postoperative period free of complications. In one case a postoperative bleeding in need of revision was noticed and a further patient developed a postoperative thrombosis of the reconstructed carotid artery. The latter patient developed a neurological deficit while still in the intensive care unit, but this receded entirely after emergency revision. Another patient developed a transient ischemic attack while in the intensive care station, too. In two cases we registered reversible pareses of the recurrent laryngeal nerve. Another patient had lesion of the mouth branch of the facial nerve.

The monitoring of cerebral function and perfusion was performed during operation by somatosensory evoked potentials (SEP) and transcranial Doppler ultrasound (TCD). 60 % of surgically treated patients (n = 15) were monitored with SEP and TCD simultaneously. In the further 40 % (n = 10) the SEP method was the intraoperative monitoring of the brain. One patient required an intraluminal shunt due to a reduction of the SEP amplitude (N20/P25) of more than 50 %. All the other operations did not necessitate a shunt.

Discussion

Surgical intervention in the presence of cerebral vessel elongations even 40 years after the first sucessful operation remains a controversy. The indication for reconstruction is the most vehemently disputed point.

The presence of clinical symptoms remains as the basis for surgical indication. Some authors, like Vollmar, consider intervention indicated mainly in symptomatic coils and kinks with angulation. Others like Leibzig see reason for intervention of kinking only in agreement with Metz grade III (angulation of elongation less than 30 degrees) excluding coiling (2, 6).

While the known classifications like Metz and Herrschaft consider the morphological criteria independent of the degree of reduction of arterial lumen (synonym: kink stenosis) due to the angulation, we introduce this parameter as another important criterium. We also consider the extent of the kink stenosis in neutral and other head positions as part of the morphological criteria to decide on the indication for surgery. According to our view, the deciding morphological parameter is not the shape or the amount of angulation on the angiography as described by Herrschaft or Metz, but the degree of stensosis caused by the kink in the position of maximum bend in the vessel.

In this way a purely spiral elongation of the internal carotid artery could result in a bend of less than 30 degrees (Metz III) in two-dimensional angiography in the absence of the significant stenosis. Furthermore, hemodynamic stenosis within coiling (particularly of the elipsoid type) can be determined. In our opinion the kink stenosis reflects the hemodynamic effect of elongated artery.

The main differences of opinion exist over indications of conservative treatment. Using the kink stenosis caused by bend in the elongation as leading parameter, we listed our views on non-indicated intervention despite symptoms:

1. C- or S-shaped elongations without angulation in neutral or functional head position
2. spiral-shaped kinkings in the absence of organic or functional stenoses
3. coilings without hemodynamic stensosis of angulations

Symptomatic carotid kinking and coiling remains an undisputed indication for surgical intervention amongst vascular surgeon. According to Leipzig only Metz grade III kinkings warrant surgical intervention, excluding coilings. End et al. considers Metz grade III with elongations to be in need of correction as purely prophylactic measure in the presence of TIA's and as palliative treatment in patients with occurred strokes (7). Vollmar considers the main indication of surgery to be symptomatic stages of the type II and III according to Herrschaft (2, 8). In our opinion the symptomatic kinking and coiling in the presence of kink stenosis is an absolute indication for surgical reconstruction. If a high-grade stenosis exists in the absence of stenosis, surgery is certainly indicated. The low-grade kink stenosis on elongation should be operated in the presence of contralateral occlusion of carotid artery. If should be noted that in the presence of atherosclerotic change inside the carotid artery a more differentiated approach is necessary.

References

1. Metz H, Murray-Lesslie RM, Bannister RG (1961) Kinking of the internal carotid artery in relation to cerebrovascular disease. Lancet 1: 424–426
2. Vollmar J, Nadjafi AS, Stalker CG (1976) Surgical treatment of kinked internal carotid arteries. Br J Surg 63: 847–850
3. Quattlebaum JK Jr, Upson ET, Neville RL (1959) Stroke associated with elongation and kinking of the internal carotid artery. Ann Surg 150: 824–832
4. Hsu I, Kistin AD (1956) Buckling of the great vessels. Arch Intern Med 150: 712–719
5. Riser MM, Geraud J, Ducoudray J, Ribaut L (1951) Dolicho-carotide interne avec syndrome vertigineux. Rev Neurol 85: 145–147
6. Leipzig TJ, Dohrmann GJ (1986) The tortuous or kinked carotid artery: pathogenesis and clinical considerations. Surg Neurol 25: 478–486
7. End A, Ehrmann L, Wimberger (1988) Die operative Therapie des Carotis-Kinkings – Retrospektive Analyse von 43 Fällen. VASA Suppl. 23: 241–243
8. Herrschaft H (1968) Zerebrale Durchblutungsstörungen bei extremer Schlingenbildung der A. carotis interna. Münch Med Wschr 110: 2694–2699

Author's address:
K. Ktenidis, MD
Dept. of Vascular Surgery
General Hospital Cologne-Porz
Urbacher Weg 19
51149 Köln, Germany

Redo-carotid surgery – indication, technique, results

K. Balzer

Department of Vascular Surgery, Evangelical Hospital Muelheim on the Ruhr, Germany

Introduction

Today an operation on the carotid artery represents a normal standard operation, the importance of which as a stroke prophylaxis has been proved by extensive, far-reaching international studies. The NASCET-study has ended – at least from the vascular surgical point of view – the long-lasting discussion of whether or not surgical interventions make sense. Amazingly the results of the NASCET- and the European trial are in agreement with those of Vollmar and my own reviews based on retrospective studies.

The indication for a carotid reconstruction continues to refer to the well known four-stage classification, whereby the indication in the asymptomatic stage must be judged carefully, as the rate of morbidity clearly is lower than the rate of mortality. The part of patients being operated on during stage I has diminished significantly in the past 12 years, but tends to be increasing currently. This is also true for redo-carotid surgery. Asymptomatic recurrent stenoses have rarely been operated in the last 10 years. Most redo operations (~ 65 %) were performed during the last 12 years and reflects the correlation with improved postoperative diagnostic management. The carotid surgery is negatively influenced by a number of postoperative neurological deficits extending to cerebral coma and death, which depend on the stage of the basic disease. Nevertheless, there are three more factors of influence: 1) indication for operation; 2) the operative technique; and 3) type of arteriosclerosis.

Reasons for recurrent stenoses

The carotid artery occlusion, which occurs as an immediate postoperative consequence or within a few days later, is mostly a technical fault. It may be caused by a floating intimal flap, a persisting ledge, or by a fold formation which protrudes into the vascular lumen. The firm, straight course of the vessel must be restored, either by internal plication of the back wall or by resecting of an entire segment of the vascular wall. The early postoperative occlusion will not be handled at this point. Fortunately not every operative fault leads to an occlusion, but more to alterations in the carotid bifurcation, which are responsible for later stenosis. There are three principle reasons causing a recurrent stenosis after carotid reconstruction, whereby the importance of the basic disease must be clearly pointed out: 1) the operative technique; 2) the intimal hyperplasia; and 3) the progressive basic disease.

A retrospective estimation of the different reasons is not possible concerning all cases, but a critical analysis is necessary. To follow-up on this problem, we have analysed our patients from 1974 to 1988 retrospectively based on clinical examinations. The redo-operations were investigated analysing the question of frequency, reasons for recurrent stenoses, and other postoperative complications.

Frequency of recurrent stenoses after carotid endarterectomy

In a retrospective study including 934 patients with 1289 operations, the Doppler ultrasound findings showed a high rate of recurrent stenoses, from 3 to 15 %. During the same period of time, reiterated transitoric-ischaemic-attacks (TIA) which could be observed on the operated side were 4 %, and completed strokes in the depending cerebral region of the operation were 3 %. In total we found a rate of TIA and stroke of 6.5 %, but the percentage of restenoses was more than double that value. It must be kept in mind that < 50 % of the symptomatic patients were found in the group of re-stenoses. The fact thing should be mentioned, however, that re-stenosis turned out to be more often symptomatic if a contralateral stenosis had been developed. That is why a prophylactic operative correction of the stenosed contralateral carotid is indicated when the degree of the stenosis rises. Certainly the transcranial Doppler may help to discover intracranial steal phenomena and neurological disorders caused by diminished blood flow leading to an indication for operation on time. According to the lifetable-analysis, an incidence for neurological disorders of 0.5 % at stage I and II, and 2 % at stage III and IV can be observed. For both groups this means a lower morbidity than mortality.

By examination with Doppler-ultrasound on the carotid artery we found that during a period of 3 years a re-stenosis may disappear spontaneously if it is caused by intimal hyperplasia whereas a similar percentage of re-stenosis has to be added. The re-stenosis rate will remain at 15 % during the following 3 years. After that time stenotic changes will occur less often around the operated carotid artery. These alterations are described in the literature as late re-stenoses, resulting from the progressive basic disease, whereas the early alterations most likely turn out to be intimal hyperplasia, which may also be progressive after the same 3 years. Only quite rarely do re-stenoses occur after 3 years postoperatively. More frequently anastomotic aneurysms of the patch plasty may be found, which appear by means of Doppler findings as a so called relative stenosis.

It can be stated that a recurrent stenosis is not identical to a repeated cerebrovascular insufficiency. On the contrary, it can be proved that in most cases re-stenoses develop asymptomatically. This is because of the development on the intimal hyperplasia, which results in a hard but smooth narrowing of the vessel not leading to embolisation and is mostly responsible for the postoperative neurological deficits. As the narrowing slowly increases, a sufficient collateralisation is possible. Attention must be payed to the external carotid artery, in which high percentage of 25 to 30 % a re-stenosis may occur after insufficient endarterectomy. This may also lead to consequences in the internal carotid artery, which could be stenosed or occluded.

A correlation of recurrent stensoses and stages of cerebrovascular insufficiency was not possible. That is also true for the risk factors and for adjuvant medication such as aspirin or warfarin. Neither the type of the arteriosclerosis nor the time of the operation is of any importance for the development of re-stensosis.

Operative treatment

In the last 23 years (1972–1994) more than 8800 operations on the carotid artery were performed, of which 236 have been redo-operations. Of 43 patients from other hospitals, 16 redo-operations were performed due to an infected patch-plasty, and 20 due to anastomotic aneurysm. Our own patients accounting for the remaining 157 with recurrent stenoses were operated on. Of those 108 were in symptomatic stages. This figure is equivalent to a little more than 1 % therefore representing an extremely low rate. This does not give a true reproduction of the relations. It often occurs that without observation an occlusion develops from a re-stenosis. Postoperative asymptomatic occlusions occurred almost twice as much in about 2 % of all cases. Half of this proportion was symptomatic. As a consequence symptomatic re-stenoses and occlusions are rarely seen. However, to our knowledge, a stroke occurred 5 times among our patients having been caused by a postoperative carotid occlusion. Also ophthalmological disorders such as venous stasis retinopathy may be due to carotid re-stenosis or occlusion.

Altogether the real frequency of a redo-operation is about 2.6 % in relation to all operations. This is in agreement with other studies and means that only every 6th patient has to undergo an redo-operation according to Doppler findings. The examinations of the redo-procedures regularly showed for the first months an intimal hyperplasia and very rarely arteriosclerotic changes. Later on, this relation changed. Usually, a renewed endarterectomy can be done with a patch-plasty. In some cases, however, an interposition of the vessel by using venous or synthetic material has to be performed.

The histological findings did not show any irregularity compared to other operated vessels. The pathologist was not able to explain the reasons for the recurrent stenoses. An increasing frequency was noted concerning the re-stenosis with haemodynamic efficacy around the tacked intimal ledge. It must be assumed that the suture may induce a proliferation of the intimal layer. This is true for the conventional technique only. In cases of the eversion endarterectomy we rarely found re-stenoses (0.8 %). Here the stenosis was usually found in the common carotid artery, probably because of insufficient exposure of the arteriosclerotic changes in this vessel.

The results of the surgical treatment were satisfying: we observed three cerebral comas and three strokes with permanent neurological deficit, which results in a higher risk than the first operation (4.2 %). The incidence of nerve injuries is quite high: eight times the hypoglossal nerve, four times the recurrent nerve, twice the glossopharyngeal nerve, and once the accessorial nerve were injured. Two patients suffered from several nerve injuries. This increased risk means that a redo-operation should be performed by an experienced and highly skilled vascular surgeon.

It is necessary to pay attention to other vascular regions, which may also be affected by the basic disease. We found an anastomotic aneurysm in a patient who was treated at another hospital. The reason for renewed neurological disorders was a stenosis on the medial cerebral artery. We performed an extra-intracranial bypass from the subclavian artery to the medial cerebral artery, with the result the patient is to this day asymptomatic.

Conclusions

Redo-surgery on the carotid artery applies a technically difficult operation with an increased risk. The indication therefore has to be put very carefully. The surgical treatment must be done by an experienced, highly skilled vascular surgeon. In most cases the intimal hyperplasia is responsible for the re-stenosis and only in a few cases is the reason the progressive basic disease. Most likely, these are the cases which demand an indication for operation because of neurological symptoms. The operative technique is as important as the frequent occurrence of re-stenoses at the distal tacking suture in the conventional operative technique as is shown by the stenosis of the common carotid artery in the eversion-endarterectomy.

References

1. Trial (NASCET) investigators (1991) Clinical alert: benefit of carotid endarterectomy for patients with high-grade stenosis of the internal carotid artery. Stroke 22: 816–817
2. Vollmer J (1982) Rekonstruktive Chirurgie der Arterie. Thieme-Verlag, Stuttgart
3. Carstensen G, Balzer K (1986) Die asymptomatische Carotisstenose: wann soll – wann muß man – wann soll man nicht operieren? Langenbecks Arch Chir 369: 97–103
4. Sundt TM Jr, Whisnant JP, Houser OW, Fode NC (1990) Prospective study of the effectiveness and durability of carotid endarterectomy. Mayo Clin Proc 65: 625–635
5. The CASANOVA Study Group (1991) Carotid surgery versus medical therapy in asymptomatic carotid stenosis. Stroke 22: 1229–1235
6. Cook JM, Thompson BW, Barnes RW (1990) Is routine duplex examination after carotid endarterectomy justified? J Vasc Surg 12: 334–340
7. Carstensen G, Balzer K (1989) Occlusions of the carotid arteries. Vascular Surgery, Springer-Verlag, Berlin Heidelberg, 463–476
8. Bernstein EF, Torem S, Dilley RB (1990) Does carotid restenosis predict an increased risk of late symptoms, stroke, or death? Ann Surg 212: 629–636
9. Gagne PJ, Riles TS, Imparato AM, Lamparello PJ, Giangola G, Landis RM (1991) Redo endarterectomy for recurrent carotid artery stenosis. Eur J Vasc Surg 5: 135–140
10. Pauliukas PA, Barkauskas EM (1990) Surgeries on the carotid arteries (Operatsii na sonnykh arteriiakh). Khirurgiia Mosk 8: 90–94
11. Archie JP Jr (1991) Early and late geometric changes after carotid endarterectomy patch reconstruction. J Vasc Surg 14: 258–266
12. Park Y, el-Bayer H, Hye RJ, Stabile BE, Freischlag JA (1990) Safety and long-term benefit of carotid endarterectomy in the asymptomatic patient. Ann Vasc Surg 4: 218–222
13. Maki HS, Kruger RA, Kuchner ME (1991) The problem of recurrent stenosis following carotid endarterectomy. Wis Med J 90: 583–585

Author's address:
Dr. Klaus Balzer
Chefarzt der Gefäßchirurgischen Klinik am Evangelischen Krankenhaus
Wertgasse 30
45468 Mülheim an der Ruhr, Germany

Emergency carotid surgery – guidelines for surgical treatment

N. Doundoulakis

Department of Vascular Surgery, "Red Cross" General Hospital Athens, Greece

Carotid surgery has been the last but most controversial field of vascular surgery. Although carotid pathology and brain ischemia have been associated since the era of Ippocrates, the history of carotid surgery goes back only 30 years. The realization that surgical intervention can at last prevent the ever fearful stroke made carotid surgery one of the commonest procedures of vascular surgery. However, many physicians kept their skepticism about the whole subject and the questions of unnecessary or, even worse, harmful procedures were raised. The need for carefully planned and conducted trials as far as the indications and the accepted outcome are concerned was obvious. The results of these trials (5, 15) define some universally accepted indications for surgery, such as tight stenosis of internal carotid of 75 % or ulcerated plaque, but failed to answer other questions. One of these is the optimum treatment of acute cerebral ischemia and the role of emergency carotid surgery. On this subject the experience worldwide is limited and virtually every carotid surgeon has developed his own policy based mainly on his experience.

Natural history

Emergency carotid surgery almost always follows acute carotid occlusion. In rare cases carotid surgery can be considered for rapidly deteriorating neurological deficit due to crescendo TIA's or progressing stroke. The cause of acute carotid occlusion is mainly thrombosis of a stenotic atherosclerotic lesion at the carotid bifurcation. Other causes are thrombosis after arteriography, after carotid endarterectomy, dissection as in fibromascular dysplasia, trauma, radiation arteritis and hypercoagulable states, i.e., due to oral contraceptives.

Carotid occlusion may result in a variety of symptoms, i.e., death, acute profound stroke, moderate stroke, mild stroke, TIA or no symptom at all. Fields and Lemak (6) in a study of 6535 patients found that 16 % (1040) of them had one or both carotids occluded, the incidence of bilateral occlusion being 1.3 %. Of these patients 72 % presented with some degree of neurological deficit. In a study by Thomson JE (19) in 1968 from 94 patients with total occlusion 71 (75 %) had frank stroke and 34 of them had profound stroke (36 %). In another study, Hafner states that carotid occlusion will result in serious stroke and/or death in 1/3 of the cases, in a mild or moderate stroke in another 1/3 and the last third will experience no symptoms (8). The above findings are more or less confirmed by many other studies. It is obvious that there is a major association between carotid occlusion and stroke. Stenotic lesions can sometimes result in a rather unusual severity of symptoms presenting as crescendo TIA's (succession of TIA's that become more severe or more frequent) or progressing stroke (neurological deficit that has progressed over a period of 24 h or more) (14). The result of these conditions is usually a frank or profound stroke.

Diagnosis

We can suspect a carotid occlusion in any case with acute mild or profound stroke. In some cases the disappearance of a previously known cervical bruit is a sign of occlusion. However, carotid bruits can be heard in up to 6 % of carotid occlusion. Duplex scan is a simple and reliable method of diagnosis, although in certain cases of occlusion may be misleading (2). The gold standard remains the arteriogram. Recent development of diagnostic methods such as MRI and CT scan angiography can be of value in the near future (4, 10). However, we must consider the time and the facilities needed for these diagnostic procedures not to mention the associated risks. As far as the brain image is concerned, MRI and CT scan can provide all the necessary information.

Surgical treatment

The key point is to select those patients that will benefit the most from emergency surgical treatment. The time elapsed from the onset of occlusion or symptoms and the clinical situation are the two most important factors to be considered. In most cases a patient presents to vascular surgeon after considerable time has elapsed from the acute stroke caused from carotid occlusion. We believe that in cases as this, surgery has no place as far as the occluded carotid is concerned. The contralateral carotid should be examined for an indication to proceed to operation. In a study by Thompson, patients operated for carotid occlusion after 1 to 7 days achieved a patency rate of 55 % and after 1 to 4 weeks only 20 % (18)! When we consider patients for emergency carotid surgery, we virtually refer to hospitalized patients, because this particular population is under close observation so that diagnosis and surgery can be performed in less than 24 hours. Although we regard the 24-h limit as a safe limit for operation, we emphasize the need for immediate action. In the previous mentioned study, restoration of blood was successful in 100 % when the operation was performed within 6 h and in 62 % for operation between 6 and 24 h. Although the time is the main factor for successful operation as far as the patency is concerned, there are some other factors that play a role. Patients on antiplatelet or anticoagulant treatment or those who, on arteriograms, have been known to have patent distal internal carotid artery via collaterals tend to achieve better results. The aim of the surgical treatment in these cases is to restore blood flow to arrest the progress or even to reverse neurological deficit.

As we stated at the beginning, not all patients are candidates for surgery even if we are within the time limit of 24 h. Clinical situation is of paramount importance. We believe that patients with profound or major stroke and loss of consciousness due to carotid occlusion should not be operated on. In many studies, the results from such operations are disappointing. Wylie reported operative mortality rate of 60 %, Blaisdell 42 %, DeWeese 34 %, Meyer and Thompson 20 % (1, 3, 13, 20, 21). The main cause of death in these series was intracerebral hemorrhage in the area of infarction. Although certain surgeons may feel comfortable to operate early after a stroke or even at the time of stroke, it has become common practice for most surgeons not to operate for at least 6 weeks after the event. Best candidates for emergency surgery are the patients who, after acute occlusion of carotid, develop a mild neurological deficit or a TIA. In this case, and provided that we act within 6 h, blood flow will be restored and the operation will have good result without complications. Candidates for emergency surgery can be patients without occlusion of carotid artery but with stenotic lesion that causes crescendo TIA's or progressing stroke. These patients should be put under close observation and constant neurological evaluation for 24 h and, if their situation remains unstable or shows evidence of deterioration, they then can be operated on as emergencies. A special case of emergency surgery is the occlusion of carotid artery after endarterectomy. Occlusion should be suspected in all cases who develop neurological deficit as soon as the patient wakes up or in the following hours.

Diagnostic evaluation with duplex scan and brain CT scan must be performed immediatly. If intracerebral hemorrhage is excluded and carotid thrombosis is confirmed, the patient should be taken back to the operating theater for carotid reexploration as soon as possible. The operative technique of acute occlusion of carotid artery is usual with a few modifications. The surgeon must be extremely careful in dissecting the carotid artery to avoid fragmentation of thrombus and distal embolization. Clamps should not be used before arteriotomy and removal of thrombus from internal carotid artery. The presence of brisk back bleeding indicates internal carotid patency. If there is any doubt, gentle exploration with a Fogarty catheter may be tried. The completion of the operation follows the usual method and the preference of the surgeon.

Results

The results of emergency carotid surgery vary according to the time elapsed after the onset of symptoms and the severity of neurological deficit. Emergency endarterectomy carried out for carotid occlusion in patients with major stroke carries a high mortality rate, as we saw, ranging from 20 % to 42 %. In these cases the functional result of the remainder was also disappointing. In case of emergency surgery for symptomatic stenosis with unstable neurological deficits (crescendo TIA's and progressing stroke) results are clearly better. Young, Hunter, Rob, Goldstone and Moore, Mentzer, McIntyre and others in their studies showed that emergency operation for progressing stroke carries a mean mortality of 10 %, while 89 % of patients improved (63 %) or showed no change (26 %) and 1 % worsened (7, 9, 11, 12, 17, 22). In the particular situation of emergency reoperation after carotid endarterectomy, results are not as satisfactory. In seven series collected from the literature, Painter et al. found an average mortality of 17 % (0 to 29 %). Functional improvement was noted in 61 % of the patients, a result that compares favorably with outcome of patients receiving supportive care alone (16). The main causes of death in these categories of patients are either intracerebral hemorrhage or cerebral infarction.

Our own material

In the Vascular Surgery Dept. of Red Cross Hospital of Athens, during the period 1991 – 1994, we performed approx. 300 operations for brain ischemia due to extracranial vascular lesions. Five of these patients were operated on as emergencies. Two of the patients were operated in less than 12 h after they developed mild or moderate neurological deficit following carotid endarterectomy of internal carotid artery. One patient developed a mild neurological deficit due to occlusion of carotid artery after arteriography. He was operated on 24 h later. Two other patients were admitted to the hospital with great stenotic lesion and crescendo TIA's and were operated within 48 h since their situation showed no improvement. Four patients improved while one with moderate neurological deficit after carotid endarterectomy and postoperative occlusion remained unchanged.

Conclusions

Emergency carotid surgery remains, in a way, an unexplored field that every surgeon has to go through based mainly on his own experience and instinct. The data from the literature are based on a few series with relatively small numbers and contradictory results. However, we think that we can define at least three categories of patients most likely to benefit from emergency carotid surgery, knowing before hand that in this particular subject there is no substitute for careful judgment and advanced surgical skill.

1) asymptomatic patients who have found to have developed carotid occlusion while in hospital

2) symptomatic patients with carotid occlusion who can withstand the operation provided that it will be in less than 6 h

3) symptomatic patients who present with unstable neurological deficit and progressing stroke due to carotid occlusion or tight stenosis

4) patients who developed neurological deficit after carotid endarterectomy, since emergency operation appears to be the appropriate treatment for this catastrophic complication.

Summary

Although carotid surgery is an established method for prevention of stroke in certain categories of patients, the role of emergency carotid surgery remains controversial. Data from the literature worldwide are inconclusive. The role of the surgeon remains important since his decision is based on his experience and his instinct and less on clearly define indications. The average mortality and the good functional result from emergency operation are considered less than satisfactory. However, in certain categories of patients, emergency carotid surgery seems to be well justify. Patients with mild or moderate neurological deficit − stable or unstable −, due to carotid occlusion or tight stenosis might benefit from emergency surgery provided that it will be performed in less than 24 h, preferably in less than 6 h. Finally, for patients who developed neurological deficit after carotid endarterectomy, emergency reoperation seems to be the best treatment in nearly every case.

References

1. Blaisdell FW, Clauss RH, Galbraith JG et al. (1969) Joint study of extracranial arterial occlusion IV. A review of surgical considerations. J Am Med Assoc 209: 1889–1889
2. Bornstein NM, Beloev ZG, Norris JW (1988) The limitations of diagnosis of carotid occlusion by Doppler ultrasound. Ann Surg 207: 315–
3. DeWeese JA, Rob CS, Satran R et al. (1968) Surgical treatment for occlusive disease of the carotid artery. Ann Surg 168: 85–94
4. Dillon EH, Eikelboom BC, Van Leeuwen M (1993) New imaging Modalities: Magnetic resonance and Computed Tomographic Angiography. Is conventional angiography still needed? Surgery for stroke. Greenhagh RM, Hollier LH (Eds) WB Saunders, p 63–70
5. European Carotid Surgery Trialists' Collaborative Group (1991) MRC European Surgery Trial: Interim results for symptomatic patients with severe (70 – 99 %) or mild (0 – 29 %) carotid stenosis. Lancet 337: 1235–1243
6. Fields WS, Lemak NA (1976) Joint study of extracranial arterial occlusion X: Internal carotid artery occlusion. J Am Med Assoc 235: 2734–2738
7. Goldstone J, Moore WS (1976) Emergency carotid artery surgery in neurologically unstable patients. Arch Surg 111: 1284
8. Hafner CD (1987) Totally and nearly occluded extracranial internal carotid arteries. In: Current therapy in Vascular surgery. Ernst CB, Stanley JC (Eds). Philadelphia: Decker BC, pp 46–49
9. Hunter JA, Julian OC, Dye WS, Javid H (1965) Emergency operation for acute cerebral ischaemia due to carotid artery obstruction: review of 26 cases. Ann Surg 162: 901
10. Masaryk AM, Ross JS, DiCello MC et al. (1991) 3DFT MR angiography of carotid bifurcation: potential and limitations as screening examination. Radiology 179: 797–804
11. McIntyre KE, Goldstone J (1983) Carotid surgery for crescendo TIA and stroke in evolution. In: Bergan JJ, Yao JST (ed) Cerebrovascular Insufficiency. New York: Grune & Stratton, Inc., p 213
12. Mentzer RM, Finkelmeier BA, Crosby IK, Wellons HA (1981) Emergency carotid endarterectomy for fluctuating neurologic deficits. J Vasc Surg 89: 60
13. Meyer FB, Sundt TM Jr, Piepgras DG et al. (1986) Emergency carotid endarterectomy for patients with acute carotid occlusion and profound neurological deficits. Ann Surg 203: 82–88
14. Millikan CH (1973) Clinical management of cerebral ischaemia. In cerebral vascular disease. Eight Conference, New York. MacDonnell FL, Brennan RW (eds) New York: Grune & Stratton, p 209
15. NASCET Collaborators (1991) Beneficial effect of carotid endarterectomy in symptomatic patients with high-grade carotid stenosis. N Engl J Med 325: 445–453
16. Painter TA, Hertzer NR, O'Hara PJ et al. (1987) Symptomatic internal carotid thrombosis after carotid endarterectomy. J Vasc Surg 5: 445–451
17. Rob CG (1969) Operation for acute completed stroke due to thrombosis of the internal carotid artery. Surgery 65: 862
18. Thompson JE, Austin DJ, Patman RD (1967) Endarterectomy of the totally occluded carotid artery for stroke: Results in 100 operations. Arch Surg 95: 791–801
19. Thompson JE (1968) Surgery for Cerebrovascular Insufficiency (stroke). Springfield, Ill: Charles C Thomas
20. Thompson JE, Austin DJ, Patman RD (1970) Carotid endarterectomy for cerebrovascular insufficiency: Long term results in 592 patients followed up to thirteen years. Ann Surg 172: 663–679
21. Wylie EJ, Hein MF, Adams JE (1964) Intracranial heamorrhage following surgical revascularization for treatment of acute strokes. J Neurosurg 21: 212–218
22. Young JR, Humphries AW, de Wolfe VG, Beven EG, LeFevre FA (1964) Extracranial cerebrovascular disease treated surgically. Arch Surg 89: 848

Author's address:
Nikolaos Doundoulakis, MD
"Red Cross" General Hospital
1, Athanasaki st.,
11526 Athens, Greece